YOUR DOCTOR IS NOT GOD

YOUR DOCTOR IS NOT GOD

How to be the CEO of your Health?

Aanchal Bhatia

B L O O M S B U R Y
NEW DELHI • LONDON • OXFORD • NEW YORK • SYDNEY

First published in India 2016

ISBN 978 93 859 3643 2
2 4 6 8 10 9 7 5 3 1

Bloomsbury Publishing India Pvt. Ltd
DDA Complex, LSC Building No.4
Second Floor, Pocket C – 6 & 7, Vasant Kunj
New Delhi 110070
www.bloomsbury.com

Edited by Ruchhita Kazaria

Typeset by Manmohan Kumar
Printed and bound in India by Thomson Press India Ltd.

Dedicated to Nana Ji
Late Shree Raj Narain Kapoor

'The Author has pledged her complete proceeds from this book to the charity Breathe Easy India'.

Author's Note

"Life is simple if we reflect upon nature and learn from it. People will remain healthy if they live in harmony with the healing energies of Mother Nature. The doctor of the future will hopefully be scientifically sound while being intuitively alert to the signals of nature.

Let food be thy medicine and medicine be thy food. Modern medical science is marvelous but is limited by its focus on physical means and methods of treatment. Methods imposed from outside whether they are biochemical, mechanical or surgical, they drastically disrupt the body's self-regulatory functions and make it vulnerable to toxins and debilitations. By focusing on relieving short-term symptoms, one ignores the underlying root of the illness, which is exponentially detrimental to curing oneself of one's illness.

We humans are an integrated product of mind, body, intellect and soul imbued with consciousness and a potential to transcend physical limitations. Modern medicine thus shall have to be reinvented and realigned to this fact of nature."

– Late Shree R.N. Kapoor

I remember my Grandfather (Nanaji) making me type this letter, which he was writing to Narendra Modi, who was then the Chief Minister of Gujarat. It was Nanaji's dream to set up an integrated centre of excellence based on ancient wisdom and cutting edge medical technology.

Nanaji had a similar vision when he laid the foundation for the University at Chitrakoot. His words still echo in my mind, as fresh and clear as the first morning dew. Those scenes come to me in bits and pieces: the huge room filled with books and sunlight, a large oval teakwood table at the center, memories of the days when the Ayurveda department used to discuss critical cases in a round table format where specialists from all branches of modern and alternative medicine were present. He was not only an educator but also a visionary whose purpose was to bring all those specialists together and integrate them into a harmonious team. For me, this was how things were supposed to be. Life was simple until I grew up and faced the harsh realities of healthcare in India.

Along the way as I dealt with my own illness and that of my family, I realized that the path to quality healthcare in India has become blocked at worst and rocky at best. Doctors are too frequently looking after diseases rather than the patient's health. People are confused and hence they keep jumping from one specialist to another with a scattergun approach. My education as a clinical psychologist, experience in the business of healthcare, nativity to the land of Karma and Kamasutra and decision to follow Mahatma Gandhi's philosophy became the seeds for the change I want to see in the world.

In establishing Texas Medical Concierge (TMC), I pioneered a new vision of concierge medicine with telemedicine and integrative medicine at the core. I would no longer tolerate what I perceived as corruption in the medical field. Rather, I dedicated myself to following the core values represented by our family business, the Uttam group, a company that was started in 1900. These values are known as the five "C's" and include courage, competence, compatibility, communication and commitment. I created a professional medical team whose aim is to keep patients healthy, and when ill, to become their advocates in acquiring the best care, regardless of where in the world this care is required.

Awareness is the first and foremost step. Sadly, sublime surrender seems to be in our collective subconscious. But it's time to change and question the meaning of health and the process of recovering from illness. In the words of Dr Gershom Zajicek, whose work deeply inspires me, 'The proof of the pudding lies in eating.' So too does the proof of well-being lies in treating.

Acknowledgements

I thank the Indian healthcare industry –which disgusted me and angered me so much –that I had to step up and write this book. The first seed of confidence was planted by Adam Kaufman, who expressed his trust in my capability and passion for patient advocacy. Many thanks to him. I express my deepest gratitude to Dr. Mark Tager – as a successful author himself, he was my backbone and mentor.

I thank Harsh Agarwal, without whom this book would not have been possible. He structured my vision into concrete thoughts and supported me word by word, and chapter by chapter. I will never forget those sleepless nights and festivals that we sacrificed together to make this book a reality. I also thank Nilofar Currimbhoy who kept guiding me at every step of this journey. My deepest regards to my spiritual Guru – Shree Shivendra Nagar and his wife Shree Prem Lata Nagar.

My deep appreciation goes to members of the Texas Medical Concierge team. Dr. Sneha Krishnan, for all her medical expertise and inputs. Dr. Anwar Taqveem, Dr. Himanshu Mahajan, Dr. Naveen Sanghwan for being my medical detectives. Akant Kumar and Karen Duarte for the research. Anupam Kumar and Sunil Rampore for the illustrations and graphics. Dicky M Eric for taking on the entire extra load at work while I was obsessed with this book. Manjeet Kaur and Yogita Gauba for all the administrative support.

I am grateful to Aditi and Niren Choudhary for introducing me to Bloomsbury, a publishing house with a soul. I will never forget the day I met Praveen Tiwari. We both had tears in our eyes in memory of Aisha.

I am indebted to my mother Shikha Kapoor Honawar; my maternal grandmother, Shanta Kapoor; my mother in law, Sudha Bhatia; and my sister, Aveena Malhotra; – all of whom were super excited and super supportive at the highest levels. Thanks to Rahul Malik for exercising with me at obscure hours due to a crazy schedule. I am ever so grateful for the support extended by sons Ashvath and Aaryaman, whose time I robbed to complete this in record time. And finally my husband and best friend, Karan Bhatia; I am blessed to have him beside me each step of the way, no matter how hard, easy or crazy it is.

Dear Luke and Rachel

Thought you may find
this interesting as a
dip into read?
It was given to me by a
lady who supports a
charity giving children in India
ENT treatments.

A xxxx

Contents

Foreword

There is an aspect of well-being that is difficult to quantify, but impossible to ignore. It is *passion*, a force rooted in conviction, and expressed without reservation. Like the invisible draw of a magnet, passion pulls people toward ideas and new ways of interacting. Passion is the prerequisite for effective leadership. No great movement has ever been successful without it.

Two years ago when I met Aanchal Bhatia at an Entrepreneur's Organization (EO) conference, I felt the pull of the magnet.

It is only now that I finally understand not just her quest – to change the healthcare system in India – but the reasons behind it. These reasons are spelled out in *Your Doctor is Not God*. Her passion was informed by early childhood experiences of misdiagnosis, and frustration with an inability to get appropriate medical care for loved ones. Her skills were built through training in psychology.

These personal experiences, however, were only kindling for the fire that was already within her.

She turned her attention to a problem that is as clear as the nose on our faces – assuming we are not outside looking into a mirror when we attempt to see our reflection: air pollution and the consequences for human lungs. The world pumped out nearly 40 billion tons of CO_2 last year, with India contributing 2.5 billion of them. But it's not just the CO_2. It is the oxides of nitrogen and sulfur, the carbon monoxide, the volatile organic compounds, toxic metals, ammonia, particulates . . . the toxic brown haze that hovers over India's major cities as an illness-inducing stew.

Realizing that numbers alone rarely move people to action, Aanchal tells the story of the victims of this environmental insult. In the pages that follow, you will find heartfelt stories of patients, both young and old, who suffer from the spectrum of lung disease: from chronic asthma, to COPD (chronic obstructive pulmonary disease), to lung cancer. With the support of the Uttam Group, a hundred year old company that provides life-saving oxygen to hospitals, she founded "Breathe Easy," a non-profit whose mission is to generate awareness, and to fight for cures, for India's lung disease epidemic.

For the last 40 years I have been both an observer of and a participant in the bipolar swings of healthcare delivery. Although my primary experience has been in the United States, many of the dynamic forces that shaped the U.S. experience are germane to other countries. The United States has witnessed the pendulum swing between two positions: one dominated by physicians, the other ruled by the payors of care. In the best of worlds, allowing well trained, well meaning physicians to care holistically for patients, and providing these physicians compensation commensurate with their efforts, provides satisfactory outcomes for both doctor and patient. Unfortunately, without oversight, some physicians may abuse the privilege and provide inappropriate testing and unnecessary procedures, to the detriment of the patient. In the pages of *Your Doctor is Not God*, you will find examples of both ends of the physician spectrum.

The insertion of insurance – either private or government – gatekeepers takes the pendulum in the opposite direction. While costs may be contained, patients may not receive quality care in a timely fashion. Payment for procedures may be limited, or gatekeepers may delay or deny payment. Of course, the greatest gatekeeper – and an issue facing many emerging economies including India – is simply access to affordable care, an issue that is beyond the scope of this work.

In the dialog between physician and payor in the United States, a third voice began to insert itself. It was in 1999 that the Institute of Medicine – a non-profit, non-governmental organization founded under the congressional charter of the National Academy of Sciences – issued its breakthrough report on how to fix an increasingly dysfunctional system.

Crossing the Quality Chasm set out six aims for changing the healthcare system. At the heart of the report was the dictum that healthcare must be patient-centered.

No longer were physicians to just dictate treatment, rather, decision-making was to be a shared responsibility. The physician was encouraged to take several steps down from his or her pedestal and look eye to eye with patients whom they would empower with knowledge and treatment options.

This change in medical mindset came at a time when other forces stoked the flames of medical consumerism, which began to impact thinking about health. While stirrings came as early as the 1970's, the rising tides of "alternative" medicine started to take hold in consumers' consciousness. Demand for natural cures, interest in body-mind-spirit treatment, herbs, meditation, acupuncture, Ayurveda, yoga . . . many of which are traditional in India, but "alternative" in the U.S., found their way into the popular culture. Physicians themselves were not immune to these beliefs.

Because quality is defined as meeting or exceeding the need of consumers, small numbers of physicians started reorienting their practices to meet this growing interest in natural health treatments. We see evidence of this shift today in the increasing number of healthcare practitioners who speak of 'holistic' and 'integrative health.' We also are seeing an increased appreciation for individual precision medicine, as evidenced by a 'functional' approach and its concern for identifying root causes of illness.

The winds of healthcare change are picking up speed in India, as well. In creating a new experience in health care, Texas Medical Concierge (TMC), Aanchal, along with her extensive team of clinicians and support staff, have also tried to bridge the chasm. In addition to the holistic and integrative aspects of their healthcare model, TMC provides help and direction when people need it most, when they are in crisis.

You will be moved by the stories in *Your Doctor is Not God*, but you will also find a practical guide to navigating the complex, ever-changing, multi-dimensional system of healthcare in India. In the pages ahead, you will be exposed to a new prescription for Indian healthcare, and taken on a journey where you will be swept away by passion, armed by knowledge, and empowered by choice.

Mark J. Tager, MD
San Diego, California
December, 2015

ONE

My Awakening

JUNE 1991

"Darling you have Asthma..." Said Dr Nazli Siddiqui – the soft spoken, loving and gentle doctor at Lawrence School Sanawar. "...And by the way, congratulations for breaking the school swimming record!"

I will never forget that day. I was breathless after the swimming gala; but unlike other swim meets, the breathlessness not only stayed with me, it got worse.

The macho Sanawarian boys put me on a stretcher and rushed me to the hospital, teasing me,

> *"Aanchal, you are such a skinny girl! Such a glucose patient huh!"*

When the doctor broke the news to me, my eyes instantly filled with tears, while I lay in the hospital bed. I did not understand what it really meant, but I understood that I had a label and a condition that I would live with for my entire life.

Today, after being through a series of personal and professional experiences in the world of medicine, I am finally able to join pieces of the jigsaw puzzle. A puzzle that began in an Indian army cantonment town called Mhow – an acronym for Military Headquarters of War.

Born to young parents, who took me out everywhere they went in the open army *Jongha*, I ended up getting pneumonia. While I recovered in short order, I developed a persistent cough when I was 10 years old. I was then told by my family that I had to take certain capsules for the next few months as I had tuberculosis. I was informed that I cannot miss a single dose because this course of medicines can only be taken once in a lifetime! I have very faint memories of that time, but I remember feeling very numb and fearless. I understood I had a life-threatening disease and this closeness to death gave me the power to become fearless.

Very soon after the diagnosis, I went away to a boarding school and my cough seemed to have settled, but of course, it was not the end of the story. Two years later, I remember waking up in an Army hospital room vomiting some black dreadful stuff – anesthesia. They had just chopped off my tonsils in the hope of curing my *seasonal* cough.

The problem never seemed to be resolved until Dr Nazli guided me out of the maze by telling me that I had asthma, not tuberculosis or tonsillitis! That was my first experience of being wrongly diagnosed, but back then this was not at all a big deal, as life was moving way too fast! I had bigger issues at hand – adjusting to boarding school life which I loved, but had challenges posed by freedom, puberty, my rebellious behaviour, poor grades, my parent's marital issues and so much more.

This was probably my first experience with the medical world. The feelings were buried in my subconscious, only to be acknowledged 24 years later when I sat down to start writing this book.

NOVEMBER 2008

Around the day when the Mumbai Taj was attacked by terrorists, a bomb burst in our lives too. My husband's father was rushed to the emergency room in New Delhi.

His problem began in 2007 when he started having issues with walking and would find it difficult to stand up if he had been sitting for a long time and felt stuck. We took him to an orthopedic doctor who did a gazillion tests and informed us that he had diabetic neuropathy and he would need injections in his spine.

We followed this treatment with no success. In fact, his symptoms worsened. Papa would tilt on his chair and remain in an angular position. We then noticed that he was becoming a little absent-minded and hence, we went to a neurologist who again couldn't give any concrete reasons. When one fine day, papa didn't come out of the loo, Karan, my husband, broke into it and found papa in no position to stand up.

We did not know what to do since my mother in-law

was his primary caregiver and was out of town. I decided to write down all the symptoms. I asked around for references for a neuro doctor, not knowing that there is a difference between a neurologist and a neurosurgeon. I just wanted someone who was renowned and closer to our home, and would see us that very day.

We landed at Dr Sogani's residence cum clinic, which happened to be located just two houses away from our family home. When we arrived for our 9 PM appointment, I handed the sheet of paper with the symptoms I had jotted down to him along with the scans. Being a clinical psychologist, I was aware of some medical terminologies like issues with gross motor functions, gait and cognition; plus a couple of others which I penned down.

No, papa did not have diabetic neuropathy. He had an even more severe condition called normal pressure hydrocephalus (NPH), which occurs when cerebrospinal fluid (CNS) collects in the brain and is unable to escape. We were informed that the condition was surgically correctable and, from the brain scans, it had existed for the past few years. But no one had referred us to a neurosurgeon before.

We decided to get the surgery done and upon admission to the hospital, we were supposed to select a team of doctors to get a clearance for surgery. So we chose a neurologist, psychologist, urologist, endocrinologist, internist, and a pulmonologist.

Surprisingly, the neurologist, Dr Suri, refused to accept the diagnosis of NPH since he was not a surgeon.

This caused us and papa a lot of anguish. I decided to confront Dr Suri; after all I was so confident after my three days of Google search, and assumed that my knowledge was superior to his decades of medical study and experience.

"Dr Suri, if it's not NPH, can you please tell me what it is?" He did not have an answer for me. However, I finally got a diagnosis of dementia out of him. So, the next logical question was:

"Then what is the cure for dementia?" He replied bluntly:

"There is *no cure as such*" I was baffled. I was not certain if this was because of his intellectual rigidity or just poor diagnosis. In hindsight, I was put in a spot to make a decision with very little medical information.

I told him very clearly that papa has zero quality of life. It was as if he is in a daze – a man who loved Urdu poetry and writing, was incapable of comprehending it now. He was physically dependent and homebound. Moreover, according to Dr Sogani and Google, papa had a condition that was palpably reversible. Why in the world would I not take a chance?

Much against Dr Suri's wishes, we got papa operated on the following morning. The result was a miracle. For us it was a miracle; we had papa back after two years. He could read and write. He was happy reciting poems in hospital; it was a fairytale but this fairytale did not last for long. Just a couple of weeks post the surgery, he woke up at night to go to the toilet. Somehow, he suddenly slipped and banged his head against a corner. Blood gushed out from his head and my mother in-law screamed for my husband Karan!

We came rushing down, put papa in the car, and rushed to Apollo Hospital. There we got him stitched up and got some brain scans done and found out that the shunt placed in his brain, to drain the fluid out, was blocked. This meant repeating the surgery, and papa could not bear to hear the mention of this; he simply broke down.

This was the first time Karan saw his hero crumble. Although the second surgery was successful, papa was not the same person. He started becoming very depressed. We tried our best to be around him all the time, cheer him up, and started psychiatric medication and psychotherapy sessions. We did everything we could until the fateful day!

That dreadful November 2008 evening, papa seemed to be a bit unusual at home. Now being a Bhatia, he had all the metabolic disorders which the Bhatias of North West Frontier are genetically predisposed to – including hypertension, diabetes and cardiac diseases. Not taking things lightly, we rushed him to a hospital which was amongst the best hospitals in town. When they told us there is nothing wrong in the reports, we shifted him to Apollo where his treating neurosurgeon, Dr Sogani was located.

He reached the hospital, ate dinner, and seemed fine to us and the resident doctors on duty. But he was not fine. He was in a preictal phase – a phase which precedes a stroke, but went unnoticed. He did have a stroke early next morning, and while trying to treat him, suddenly his kidneys started failing; he had suffered a massive heart attack. We did not know what was going on behind those ICU curtains. Papa was now in a coma.

My husband Karan is the only child of his parents, so saving his father was my sole purpose and getting him back from coma was my mission. Our goals were aligned as were our lives. After all, we worked in the same business, had the same professional aspirations, and had two incredible sons who looked up to their grandfather. I had fallen in love with Karan at the age of 15, married him at the age of 21, and started working for the family business at the age of 29. So, I understood that for Karan, his father was his heartbeat; papa was the person responsible for Karan's deepest pains and highest pleasures. Karan was emotionally broken. He could not understand how someone like his father who harmed no one in his life, lived with nobility and generosity, could be in this position? Papa was karmically not supposed to be punished, because he was a good soul! Nothing made sense.

We were in a complete frenzy and consulted doctors in Mumbai, Cleveland and Norway. Through this harrowing experience, the worst moment occurred when we were thrown into a situation where we had to massage a bunch of doctors' egos. Although there was an entire entourage of specialists plus three family doctors looking after him, everyone was working in silos. We thought we had the best doctors in the country, and in fact we did; but little did I realise that they were not a team. Little did I realise that I was the ringleader of this circus, constantly looking for answers on the internet or through other non-credible sources!

Stepping up as the practical one in the family, I decided that I will move papa back home even if it meant setting up an ICU at home; and we did exactly that. I trained myself to become a nurse, made spreadsheets based on the hospital protocols, procured all the equipment and supplies, and appointed a medical care team. We left no stone unturned and created an ICU at home. His bedside was piled high with surgery reports and x-rays. Round the clock, our medical team attended to him, but all in vain. He was in a coma with his entire body paralysed. Only his eyes would open but they were devoid of any expression. My soul used to weep seeing Karan live through his worst fears.

I was looking for a miracle, and at that point, I was too blinded to notice the dysfunctional healthcare system in India. We had been supplying gases and laying medical gas pipelines for hospitals for more than 45 years, so we were not new to the healthcare world. I realise now that we did not understand to what level a hospital stoops to make money or understand how the hospital's money-making machinery worked. I was also unable to realize the reasons why we were granted a discharge from the ICU after two months; it's now that I understand that it was because all his infections were hospital acquired!

We lost papa in March 2009, but that day, a seed was sown with a latent desire in me to fight the system and to stand up for what is right.

* * *

It took us a year to bounce back to normalcy and personally, it was the worst year of our lives. We had sent our 10-year-old son away to a boarding school in England. At work, I had launched a new product OxyGo, a portable oxygen kit which was facing resistance from doctors. Things could not be worse, everything was falling apart, and life seemed like an uphill climb.

Karan would tell me to stop focussing on individual OxyGo sales and concentrate on the larger institutional sales business where we supplied to the armed forces and multiple specialty gas companies. I would argue with him and say that I feel proud that our Indian soldiers have the best and lightest oxygen cylinder on their backs but what about the Indian patients?

Hospitals in India still use World War II cylinders made out of iron – they are rusted, heavy, and impossible for the patients to operate by themselves. Worst of all, most people on long-term oxygen therapy had to be home-bound.

To my utter disgust and naivety, I was told by the doctors that they were not incentivised enough to prescribe these portable lightweight aluminum cylinders because they were too inexpensive compared to oxygen concentrators. Oxygen concentrators are electronic machines that need to be plugged in and placed on the bedside; typically, patients on these machines would be almost animal-like on a 15-meter leash. Using a portable cylinder would mean freedom; it would mean getting a glimpse of their life back. Corruption at this level made me feel sick in my gut!

I know I live in India and I am not Gandhi. There are numerous occasions where greasing palms is the norm. It makes life and business less complicated. Whether it's that ₹10 to the parking lot attendant who has made a business around unauthorised parking lots or it's offering commissions for issuing a driving license. For most projects, you need the blessings of a gatekeeper.

Everyone's threshold for corruption is different. But for me, commercial interests coming in the way of life and death are not okay! Paying the mortuary to release your loved one's dead body is not okay! To confine a person to his bed for the rest of his life is not okay! To build an entire healthcare system around sickness and not health is not okay!

I know I could not beat the system so I wanted to fight it in a constructive manner. I discussed this issue with a senior pulmonologist in Delhi – Dr R. K. Mani.

He casually remarked, "*Aanchal, why don't you start a support group?*"

I went back and discussed the thought with my business partner and dear friend Rebecca Rix from the UK. She jumped at the idea of patient empowerment. Becky had lost her father to emphysema, which is a chronic lung disease involving inflammation of the air sacks. Destiny had brought us together when we started our partnership firm to sell consumer products and services which our parent company, the Uttam Group, produced the components for.

We started a Home Oxygen Therapy Service and started retailing OxyGo, portable oxygen cylinders, through pharmacies and other distribution channels. It did not make us millionaires but we both had tears in our eyes each time someone called us and thanked us saying we impacted their lives in a major way.

I cannot verbalise the joy of a bedridden father who was able to attend his daughter's wedding, thanks to OxyGo.

We were changing lives and it was just the beginning. Today we have touched over a million lives.

* * *

Without a plan, Becky and I decided to take the plunge and start a not-for-profit organisation and a patient support group. We went to meet one of Dr Mani's patients–Mr Tilak Dhar, a prominent businessman suffering from Chronic Obstructive Pulmonary Disease (COPD) in New Delhi. He had his entire life sorted and organised around his illness, and we were so impressed to meet him. Forget giving him support, he was such an inspiration for us that we felt empowered to start what we named *Breathe Easy India*. We started in October 2012 by holding our first support group meeting at his home. We invited a pulmonologist and patients and families of those suffering from lung diseases.

We then went to several other doctors to tell them about the success of our first support group and requested them to help us recruit more patients. Now again, to my utter horror, they declined this request saying:

"*All this sounds great but my patient will end up going to another doctor*." Hence, we decided that we would hold awareness events for each doctor's patients in their practicing hospital itself.

There was a brand new hospital in town where we decided to have a mega awareness event. This was a turning point in our careers because we did not realise what a national problem COPD was. It was, and still is, the third leading cause of death in India, after heart attacks and strokes. Very often lung disease causes stroke and heart disease, so indirectly it is the biggest killer. And we were the first not-for-profit organization focussed on respiratory diseases! We were surprised but determined to create a respiratory revolution.

We started putting together these events and met three beautiful souls as a result. The first was Dia Mirza; she is a popular Bollywood actress known to our family. We called Dia to tell her that we want to raise awareness about lung diseases and COPD. She asked me to describe more about COPD, and as I spoke, Dia asked me to keep going on, and then she suddenly revealed:

"*Oh my God Aanchal I think my Mom has COPD! What should I do*?" She visited a pulmonologist, and to her shock, she discovered that her mother's lungs were like that of a 106-year-old person! Her mother quit smoking that very day. Dia's life was touched directly by Breathe Easy India and she has been an ardent supporter ever since.

* * *

JANUARY 2015

The second remarkable lady we met was Aisha Chaudhary. At that time she was a 17 year old suffering from pulmonary fibrosis. She was born with an immunodeficiency disorder and had to undergo a bone marrow transplant as a result of which she developed the fibrosis. Aisha was the daughter of Niren Chaudhary – president of the South Asia operations of the PEPSICO brand; and Aditi Chaudhary, who is a mental healthcare worker.

I will never forget Aditi calling me up on January 23rd,

> *"Aanchal, Aisha is dying. She is consuming a cylinder every 2 hours. Please can you ensure that lack of oxygen is not the reason she dies. I don't want to hospitalise her to prolong her misery by putting her on a ventilator."*

I handed the phone to Karan and asked him to find a solution! He was concerned that a consistent supply might get difficult because of the upcoming Republic Day celebrations on January 26th and there would be roadblocks as the US President Obama was visiting as the guest of honour. Karan then had an idea:

> *"We supply mobile oxygen plant to the Indian Army for their high altitude battlefields. How about we install one in her home?"*

It was 11 PM at night; with the help of our 17-year-old son Aaryaman, Karan loaded the 100 kg plant into our SUV. Our head of cylinder-sales, plant manager and engineer – all reached; and so did an entire van full of oxygen cylinders to ensure that a consistent and uninterrupted supply of oxygen was provided to Aisha. We reached there but were pained to see Aisha gasping for breath. We set up the entire backup system and each of us dealt with our own pain silently.

Aisha had written a book, *My Little Epiphanies*. Her first copy arrived that same evening. It was going to be launched at the Jaipur Literary festival on January 27th. Aisha's older brother was cuddled up in bed with her and did not leave her side. He was reading out excerpts from her book to inspire her to fight. It was all too painful for me as an outsider. I cannot imagine the pain the immediate family must have gone through. Aisha left us forever that night. It's as if she waited to see that book.

I will never forget Aisha's words at a Breathe Easy event:

> *"Each night I would dream. I would visualise what may seem like the smallest of things. I'd imagine myself walking around the market in London with my friend. I'd dream of dancing endlessly at my cousin's wedding. I'd visualise things down to every little detail. The colour of my outfit, which song I'd dance to, the setting of the stage and my family celebrating. I dreamed of running around the garden with my two dogs. I wished that I'd get out of that wheelchair and actually walk, to my bathroom. I'd play a movie, in my mind, of all the things that seemed completely impossible in that one moment."*
>
> – Aisha Chaudhary

Till today, nine months later, I have not mustered the courage to read her book. I have an entire carton sitting in front of me, but I am not able to get started on spreading Aisha's Little Epiphanies, but I will. It's not just a matter of a few bucks that people should buy for charity, but it's an inspiration that we all could do with, and face harsh realities smiling in '*sassy*' way as Niren would put it.

Aisha was an inspiration for Dia, Becky and me. Dia and Aisha became good friends and she mourns the loss of Aisha very deeply. But she wants to keep Aisha's legend alive and one day, God willing, she will produce a film and have a daughter named Aisha.

* * *

Aisha was not the only warrior I had met in my life. The third incredible young lady who left a lasting impact on us was Neha Mehndiratta, aged 18 when we met her. She was an auto rickshaw driver's daughter who was afflicted with old pulmonary Koch's disease with bronchiectasis, bronchial hyper-reactivity that doctors diagnosed as a Type 2 respiratory failure.

Students race against time when it comes to taking and clearing their exams successfully, but for the 18-year-old Neha Mehndiratta from Delhi's Lodhi Colony area, the struggle had a whole different meaning. Neha could only hold herself for 90 minutes before violent coughs attack her again.

When I first met Neha, like a fragile baby, she was curled up in her bed. At that point, all I could do was reassure her that she would have a lifetime of free oxygen supply from us. Eventually, Aisha and Neha got to know each other. Neha's family found the greatest support in Aditi since they were both in the same boat with similar aged daughters who were dying from a lung disease. The major difference was the income level.

Neha was a fighter. She told us she wanted to die trying, and unlike Aisha – who did not want a lung transplant, she did. One of her doctors confirmed that yes, it was a possibility in her case.

Our medical concierge team contacted the only hospital in the country that had claimed to have had success with this procedure. This hospital did a video consult with us where our concierge physicians presented her case. Neha's father, Mr Raj Kumar came to our telemedicine lounge and Aditi dialed into the conference bridge by phone. This hospital confirmed to us that Neha was a candidate for bilateral lung transplant but with a very high risk; and we should arrange funds close to ₹ 30 lakh (approximately US$50,000). At that point Dr Anwar Taqweem, a concierge physician at TMC was close to tears, not able to express her frustration at the debauchery of affairs. How can they even say yes to a transplant for a girl who has latent tuberculosis, bronchiectasis and aspergillosis? For a transplant, you have to suppress the body's entire immune system, and in Neha's case, her TB would flare up. On our further probing, a global expert from Cleveland Clinic and Baylor College of Medicine, vehemently refused the idea of transplant.

Neha wanted to live, she wanted to fight. Each time I spoke to her, the only advice I could give her was to give one day at a time. She would say,

> *"Ma'am all I want is an outing. I am tired of living in this 10 feet by 10 feet room with a kitchen in one corner and a bathing area in another."*

Unfortunately, I was never able to fulfill this dying wish of hers since it meant the risk of spreading infection to others. That's also the only reason Aisha and Neha never met. We lost Neha on 15th of August – the day India got her independence. She got her independence too. She was free from her miseries.

TWO

Science and Spirituality Split

Helpless but determined to bring about a change, I decided to question everything about the core fundamentals of medicine. As scientific knowledge has a shelf-life, I began to wonder if modern medicine is approaching its expiry date. I wanted to know everything from scratch, so I engrossed myself in reading and researching about the evolution of medicine.

Medical knowledge is neither static nor absolute. Medicine as an art, and the science of healing is constantly changing. What we know today will also change, since change is the only thing that is constant.

The World Health Organization's 1948 definition of health sounds utopian. Health is defined as *a state of complete physical, mental and social well-being and not merely the absence of disease or infirmity.*

This definition often stands in contrast with the modern practice of medicine, in which a reductionistic viewpoint prevails. Physicians often will view patients as organs or disease processes. A loved one becomes a cardiac or a liver patient and the treatment remains focussed on curing that organ, or eliminating the bacteria, virus, or disease process that underlies it.

While many of the earlier practices or systems of medicine may be discredited today, it is important to look at the dynamic nature of this understanding. Our preoccupation with Western medical theories is often at the expense of spiritual truth. Being a psychologist, I have been deeply influenced by Carl Jung's theory of collective unconscious. Unlike an individual's subconsciousness, which comprises repressed experiences, the collective unconscious is something each of us is born with. One cannot acquire this strata by education or other conscious effort because it is innate. This is a sublime knowledge that we carry forward from generation to generation.

I was fortunate to be exposed to spirituality in a very liberal way, and as such, I tend to question things. My training as a psychologist makes me see trends and patterns instead of accepting things as absolute.

At the age of 11, I spent almost a year at Maharishi Mahesh Yogi's Ashram on the outskirts of Delhi. This Ashram was more like a resort as it had all the luxuries of the eastern and western world. My maternal grandfather was a part of Maharishi's core group of trustees and strategists, as a result of which, I got to spend time with many conscious souls. I learnt meditation. I met people from various parts of the world who would come, live with us at the ashram and pursue their inner spiritual journey. I was fascinated to learn the *siddhis* that the more experienced and evolved practitioners of Transcendental Meditation were able to do.

How is all this even possible? My grandfather would tell me,

"Close your eyes. Focus on the centre of your forehead between your eyes. What do you see?"

"A light.", I would tell.

"This is the power of your pineal gland. A gland that calcifies by the time we are 9-10 years old due to lack of stimulation. With meditation, you can keep this capability alive."

Nana Ji (my grandfather) was an engineer and an educationist, and his scientific interests were black holes and the God particle. He opened up my mind to see a universal similarity in human beings; a similarity that has been there since the beginning of mankind.

All ancient civilisations have left traces of evidence in their texts of how they practiced medicine. The definition of medicine might be different from what we interpret today but what has been constant is the subjective meaning of disease – that is not being at ease with yourself.

Certain knowledge, natural laws, or truths, have remained eternal. The functioning of the mind, body and spirit is a constant that remains unchanged. Over time, the most prominent philosophies in medicine are the Greek, the Chinese, the Egyptian and the Indian. Perhaps the biggest similarity of overall philosophy and approach is between Greek and Chinese medicine, since they both emphasise maintaining homeostasis or establishing equilibrium between complementary but opposite forces. All ancient healing traditions were committed to using natural medicine and treatments that allowed nature to work and strengthen the inherent constitutional resistance and recuperative powers of an organism.

Somewhere along the line, science prevailed over nature, and in the quest to live forever, this exploration lost focus. The focus turned towards disease and away from health. Looking back at this evolution can be quite fascinating to behold, and to note what our forefathers did and see where our collective unconsciousness is rooted.

EGYPTIANS HAD HOSPITALS CALLED THE "HOUSE OF LIFE"

The earliest evidence of medical evolution can be found in the Egyptian dynasty, which had a designated "House of Life" to deal with various health issues. Imhotep was the first known physician, as noted in the oldest references of medicine by the Egyptian civilisations in 2750 BCE.

EGYPTIANS WERE ALSO THE PIONEERS IN SUPER SPECIALISATION

The earliest Egyptian systems of healing also included specific healers for different types of diseases. The concept of super specialisation that we endorse now was understood and adapted very early. There is evidence of the earliest known surgeries being performed during this era. Egyptian medicine also edged towards supernatural causes and treatments.

THE CONCEPT OF ANALYSING SYMPTOMS AND CURING IS AS OLD AS 2000 BC

The tangible roots of modern medicine can be found in Mesopotamian texts, documented in 2000 BC. During this era, the concepts of diagnosis, prognosis, medical prescriptions and physical examinations were pioneered. These texts describe a list of symptoms, along with the observations and logical rules to heal.

THE FIRST MEDICAL SCHOOL WAS ESTABLISHED IN GREECE IN 700 BC

1300 years after the Egyptians first pioneered medicine, the Greek civilisation started the first known medical school around 700 BC in Cnidus. Alcmaeon, the author of the first anatomical work, is believed to have worked in this school. Ancient Greeks developed the humoral system of medicine. It was based on *restoring the balance of humours* in the body. They believed that the entire human body was filled with four basic substances known as humours. The 4 homours were yellow bile, black bile, phlegm and blood. The balance of these substances was to be maintained if health was to be restored. It was only around 400 BC that Hippocrates, who is considered *The Father of Medicine*, initiated a rational approach towards medicine. Hippocrates was the first to categorise illness further as acute, chronic, endemic and epidemic. Moreover, Hippocrates introduced terms like *exacerbation, relapse, resolution, crisis, paroxysm, peak and convalescence.*

Hippocrates believed that the balance of humours could restore health, and blood being one of the four humours, led to the common practice of bloodletting. The *bad blood,* which was the probable cause of any ailment or irregularity, had to be drained out. An overabundance of blood could also be used for diagnosis. The use of leeches to suck the blood was also prominent. Medieval practitioners would recommend leeching for an ailment as simple as a sore throat or as serious as plague.

Later, it was Herophilus (325 BC–280 BC) who worked at the medical school of Alexandria, and established the fact that intelligence is associated with brain function, while the motions and sensations are linked with the nervous system.

Ancient Roman medicine can be credited for inventing many surgical instruments like forceps, cautery, cross-bladed scissors and more.

ACUPUNCTURE AND TRADITIONAL CHINESE MEDICINE ARE AS OLD AS THE STONE AGE

From early writings, it is clear that the East viewed medicine as the study of life. The beginnings of such ancient systems of medicine like the Chinese and Indian are hard to trace. Acupuncture is believed to have been practiced since the Stone Age. The Eastern philosophy that supports Traditional Chinese Medicine (TCM) has evolved over years and been modified throughout history, since it has been largely based on accumulating observations. TCM focusses on relief through balancing energy channels through diet, tai chi exercises, and acupuncture.

ANCIENT INDIA WAS RICH WITH DEVELOPMENTS IN MEDICINE

The ancient Indian system of medicine is based on the principles of Ayurveda. It is thought that this system of healthcare began 8000 years ago, but there is very weak and scattered information documented about its origin. Ayurveda is not focussed on the study of disease, rather it is based on a broader perspective, which is clear in the literal meaning of the word Ayurveda. *Ayu* means life and *Veda* implies knowledge, and hence, *Ayurveda* can be defined as the knowledge of life. The best part about Ayurveda is that, unlike the Egyptian systems, it clearly distinguishes itself from the supernatural or magical aspect. It is explicitly clear that Ayurveda is in no way related to Voodo, hocus-pocus or any kind of witchcraft. It simply focuses on the link that exists between the disease and the healing procedure.

Ayurveda also emphasises that it is not just knowledge which can heal. The art of healing is beyond knowledge. It is about understanding everything associated with it. Another historical Indian physician, Charaka, aptly states:

> "[1]*A physician who fails to enter the body of a patient with the lamp of knowledge and understanding can never treat*

diseases. He should first study all the factors, including environment, which influence a patient's disease, and then prescribe treatment. It is more important to prevent the occurrence of disease than to seek a cure."

Ayurveda features no instant pain relievers or antibiotics, nor does it work against the metabolism of the body. There are no corrosive inorganic substances in Ayurveda, hence, there are no documented side effects. Healthy transformation of the patient takes place gradually over time, as the body begins to come into balance.

THE INDIAN PHYSICIAN SHUSHRUTA WAS THE FIRST GREAT ANATOMY TEACHER

The first evidence of ancient Indian medicine was a surgery performed by Sushruta around 800 BC. He was believed to be the first doctor to systematically study human anatomy. His methods are detailed in his book, *Shushruta Samahita*, which explains how anatomy can be studied by using a dead body. Sushruta is also credited with introducing plastic surgery and many other significant contributions in the world of medicine.

EMBEDDED IN THE PRINCIPLES OF AYURVEDA IS YOGA

The roots of yoga can be found around 3000 BC. The earliest mentions of the meaning of yoga are in the Rig Veda which claims its origin from the Sanskrit word *yuj*, which means to unite. The union referred to here is that of the individual self-uniting with the cosmic consciousness or the universal spirit. The modern practice of yoga can be attributed to Patanjali, who wrote *Yogasutra* in 2100 BC. Patanjali explains that the human body has channels called *nadi* and centres of energy called *chakras*. Yoga is an inward journey that simplifies *all that is in creation*. It is a set of practices aimed to calm the mind, which in turn controls the body.

The core purpose of Eastern and Western approaches to health remained the same – restoring the health by maintaining balance and healing the body. Medicine was evolving in different parts of the world independently, with different thought processes and approaches.

HEALING TURNED INTO TREATING

Somewhere in the last 150 years, with the advancements in science, healing turned into treating. Life expectancy began improving in 1850. Scientifically based treatment has its own evolutionary path, a path marked by a very sharp turn that began in the middle of the 19th Century. In 1850 AD, the average life expectancy was 36.6 years; today it is around 80. It was during this time that innovative scientists, despite resistance from the clergy, pioneered new theories of life, health and disease. Examples include Charles Darwin's *Theory of Evolution* and Gregor Johann Mendel's basic principle of genetics. Other technological advancements led to some major breakthroughs in the early part of the 20th century, all of which contributed to dramatically affecting longevity. Among the advancements were:

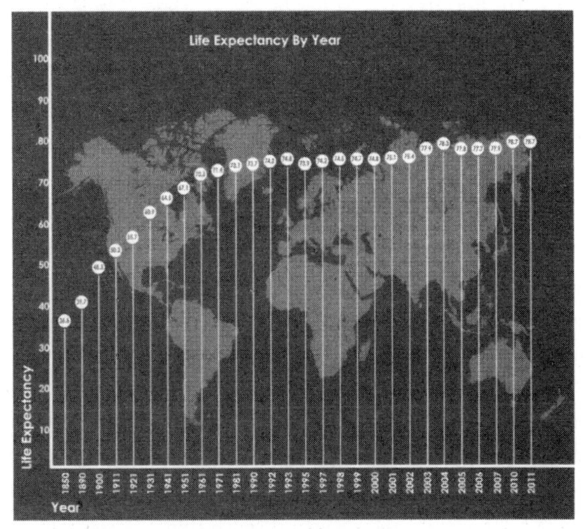

Illustration 1

1914 – Typhoid vaccine
1922 – Insulin
1928 – Antibiotic reduced post-surgical infections
1937 – Blood bank
1943 – Penicillin mass production

Along with the advances in science, other advances, related to industrialisation, helped to extend longevity. These same advances in industrialization led to a new set of diseases.

INDUSTRIALISATION HAD A MAJOR IMPACT ON THE DEVELOPMENT OF MEDICINE

The steady march of industrialisation that began in the late 18th century, took hold in the 19th century and continues today, has strongly influenced the health status. The last two centuries have witnessed important events and developments in scientific innovations as well as discoveries in varied domains. The advancements in the general modes of communication and postal services also augmented growth in medical science in all aspects.

It was a distinctive period when old ideas and conventions regarding disease control and detection gave rise to bacteriology as well as virology. The rapid development of industries gave way to diseases related to occupational hazards. Diseases of lungs, skin infections, and cancers, developed as a result of exposure to hazardous substances. For example, the match industry gave birth to jaw necrosis, a disease that was associated with workers who dealt with phosphorus. There was a sharp rise in epidemic diseases during this period.

As wars became frequent with advanced technologies, injuries became more threatening and required advanced techniques of surgical precision. As urbanisation evolved, it brought over diseases like Cholera and Typhus. Yellow fever emerged as people travelled around Europe. By 1900, pneumonia as well as tuberculosis emerged and advancements in science gave rise to antibiotic use that resulted in the serious decline of death rates.

The nature of disease changed; reason being the

development of medicine, economy and world as a whole, and by the end of 20th century, it was a different world with different expectations – for both patients and doctors.

> *"The world is round and the place which may seem like the end may also be the beginning."* – Ivy Baker Priest

This quote got stuck in my mind when we were thinking of starting a new business in Texas. I was awestruck by the Texas Medical Center, the largest medical center in the world. It is so large that it's the sixth largest downtown in the world, the third-most visited place by heads of state after the United Nations and the White House. I wanted the entire world to have access to this brilliant centre of excellence. And I wanted people at the medical centre to have access to ancient systems of medicine which were being practiced in geographical isolation.

Integrating healthcare beyond borders, we started Texas Medical Concierge to plug the gaps that I saw in healthcare. We needed to develop a system of medicine that drew upon ancient knowledge and integrated it with scientific technology.

There has been no major discovery in medicine for more than half a century. Modern technology has been the single most dramatic development in the 20th century. So why not leverage this to bring about a radical change in healthcare? What is the next stage of evolution which would rectify the current flaws in healthcare and set the scattered pieces of this puzzle right?

THREE

Rhapsody of Realities

Healthcare today is unfortunately flat lying in the ICU and needs a critical care team to defibrillate it out of its arrested state. The foundation of medical practice is shaken. Empirical sciences are caught in a paradox of crisis and opportunity. Based on the success of the advancements made in the 20th century, the only motivator driving innovation today is commercialisation. There are changes happening at multiple dimensions.

There is no doubt that these rapid scientific advancements have been the best thing that has happened to human civilisation in the last two centuries, and are the major reasons that we are living to see our grandchildren's babies. However, being cognizant of its dark side, we not only maximise the quality of this longer life, but also avoid becoming victims. Can you list the top three most common causes of death today? Chances are you'd get the first two: cardiovascular disease and stroke. But what about number three? I'll bet you'd be surprised to learn that it goes by a fancy name known as iatrogenic disease which causes 225,000 deaths per year in the US. This is death at the hands of poor decisions by physicians. Officially, according to WHO, the third leading cause of death is COPD.

"[1]*It is evident that the American medical system is the leading cause of death and injury in the United States."* Says Gary Null, who is a popular author and an American radio talk host.

To quote[2] Ido Weinberg, an assistant professor at Harvard Medical School,

"[3]The modern practice of medicine is beyond the doctor patient relationship. It is governed by several other aspects which are legal and financial. These factors sometimes are not negligible and may take precedence over medical ethics."

He asserts that the guidelines provided do not always conform to a specific patient's best interests. The prime reason here is the different structuring of reimbursements. It presents a substantial amount of payment for performing procedures than withholding on them, which poses a problem. Theoretical treatment of various stages of diseases with non-invasive methods, medicines, and other processes can occur. It is important to determine when the requisite procedures or medicines are not sufficient for treatment. This elusive arena of medicine comprises of events where making a treatment-related decision must adhere to subjective components of medicines.

Another possible reason for the onslaught of iatrogenic disease is the bewildering pace of medicine, a pace that reflects the rapid changes in our external worlds. There are changes happening at multiple dimensions. Our external world is changing so rapidly that the inner world is getting dizzy. The definition of success needs to be redefined.

This success we value today, makes us obsess with accumulating power, wealth, property and objects. We see that amidst all our success in the external world, we have accomplished little of lasting value. These problems will not be solved through new technological developments, instead, the resolution to these human problems will come only when we discover within ourselves and restore a value system based on healing and not treating.

Looking outward in this pursuit of amassing wealth by itself is a plague. I personally have no issues with commercialisation, but at what cost? Where do we draw the line? How far do we want to go from nature and its laws? How much are we willing to degrade our moral construct?

MEDICINE IS NOT PURELY SCIENCE

The practice of medicine has a strong subjective component to it and the inevitable human element which sadly is faced with the same issues that mankind faces in the 21st century.

Vanderbilt University Medical Center's chief information officer, Mr William W. Stead states that,"[4] The existing healthcare environment is characterised by intrinsic distrust, misinterpreted incentives and unnecessary competition among stakeholders.

Looking to a future that will be defined by individualised medicine, Stead suggested that tomorrow's opportunities may not be fully realised without fundamental changes in the healthcare culture. Education for health professionals is only one area that needs reform."

In my opinion, reform needs to start at a moral level. Physicians need to take a 360 degree turn and look inwards for a change. Their education is incomplete and all the outer knowledge of anatomy is incomplete without the sight of their inner eye.

> *"We should take care not to make the intellect our god; it has, of course, powerful muscles, but no personality."*
> – Albert Einstein

In the words of Albert Einstein –"[5]The further the spiritual evolution of mankind advances, the more certain it seems to me that the path to genuine religiosity does not lie through the fear of life, and the fear of death, and blind faith, but through striving after rational knowledge.

Everyone who is seriously involved in the pursuit of science becomes convinced that a spirit is manifested in the laws of the Universe – a spirit vastly superior to that of man, and one in the face of which we, with our modest powers, must feel humble. The intuitive mind is a sacred gift and the rational mind is a faithful servant. We have created a society that honours the servant and has forgotten the gift."

In the 1800's we witnessed poor medical practices. Scientific discovery of drugs that could be mass produced was possibly the single most advancement that helped in increasing life expectancy.

The pharmaceutical industry is hence dictating much of the current healthcare culture. Government can only provide a limited amount of funds and plays a limited role, since the numbers are growing.

According to an article in Forbes, "[6] For years, researchers, including one team from Tufts University and another at Eli Lilly, have estimated the cost of inventing and developing a drug at US$1 billion or more. These estimates try to exclude costs not directly related to a drug's approval and also don't allow for any comparisons between companies."

An enormous amount of money is spent on developing a drug. However, research and surveys clearly exhibit that the cost for marketing any drug is usually more than the cost that was involved for the development, sometimes even more than double.

"[7]The biggest spender, Johnson & Johnson, shelled out US$17.5 billion on sales and marketing in 2013, compared with US$8.2 billion for R&D. In the top 10, only Roche spent more on R&D than on sales and marketing.

Most of this marketing money is directed at the physicians who do the prescribing, rather than consumers. As pointed out, drug companies spent more than $3 billion year marketing to consumers in the U.S. in 2012, but an estimated $24 billion marketing directly to health care professionals."

A survey of clinical trials concluded that 90 percent of the drugs which are funded by private companies pass the approval tests while for the non-funded drugs, the data are merely 50 percent. *Money can't buy love and happiness, but it can definitely buy some desired scientific result.*

To make matters worse, drug companies are notorious for dumping drugs that are banned in developed nations onto third world countries. These drugs are available over the counter and are being taken regularly by a large population in the developing world.

A WHO report states that "[8] *For the first time in history, more than 50 per cent of the world's population lives in an urban area. By 2050, 70 per cent of the world's population will be living in towns and cities.*

The world is rapidly urbanising with significant changes in our living standards, lifestyles, social behaviour and health", says Dr Jacob Kumaresan, director of the World Health Organization's Centre for Health Development based in Kobe, Japan.

It is true that urban living offers enormous opportunities, and with these come the challenges of unhealthy urban living.

"This urbanisation that's taking place around the world is very real. But if it's people are seeking an urbanised environment out of desperation, that's not going to be helpful in the long term."
– Mick Cornett

Here are a few shocking facts that help us see things in a correct perspective. Unfortunately the data is based on American statistics due to the lack of availability and research in India.

Fact # 1 Lifestyle-related diseases top the charts

There are several diseases that occur due to stress as well as irregular lifestyle, coupled with injurious habits like drinking that take a serious toll on health and wellness. Further there are environmental challenges in cities with polluted air and water that cause diseases like cancer, diabetes and COPD with long-term exposure. Non-communicable diseases are a matter of grave concern for the medical fraternity and society as a whole.

Urbanisation and relatively better lifestyle opportunities have deviated the healthcare industry.

All leading economies in the world are spending significantly in healthcare. The statistics of patients and the amount which is being spent for them is surprising.

- 100 million people over the age of 15 in Europe suffer from a chronic disease
- US$159B are spent by European healthcare systems every year treating heart disease, pulmonary illness and diabetes
- 75 percent of chronic conditions account for more than three-quarters of US healthcare costs
- 260 million Chinese patients suffer from chronic conditions

Fact #2 The numbers don't make sense

Despite this, while considering the mathematics of healthcare, an estimated 210,000 patients are killed annually by medical errors. That's the equivalent of 10 jumbo jets crashing each week. One third of healthcare spending is spent on things that don't make people any healthier. That's US$765 billion gone in waste. Sources of waste in American healthcare are:

- Unnecessary Services = US$210B
- Excessive Administrative Costs = US$190B
- Inefficiently-delivered Services = US$130B
- Prices that are too high = US$105B
- Fraud = US$75B
- Missed Prevention Opportunities = US$55B

Fact # 3 Medicine is going digital

"[9]*Technology will revolutionise healthcare. In fact, it is already doing so. The question the industry needs to answer is how much of this change is driven by healthcare organisations themselves and how much is down to governments, patients, vendors or tech giants such as Apple, Google and Microsoft.'* – Liam Walsh, Advisory Industry Leader, Healthcare and Life Sciences, KPMG US.

- 26 per cent of US hospitals participate in social media
- 15 per cent of US hospitals were using the cloud to store images in 2013. This is expected to exceed 50 per cent by the end of 2016

- 21 per cent of US adults say they use technology to track their health data
- 500 million people around the world will use a healthcare app this year

There are approximately 76 million smartphone users in India and the figure is growing with each passing day which means India is not very far behind the US in the context of medicine going digital.

According to an article in New York Times,

> "[10]*The Company sells software that allows doctors to type in a patient's symptoms and, in response, spits out a list of possible causes. It does not replace doctors, but makes sure they can consider some unobvious possibilities that they may not have seen since medical school."*

An ironic take on digitisation can be observed in your inability to read a doctor's handwriting and prescription, but your clear reading of his neatly typewritten bills.

Fact # 4 The medical industry is a cash cow

A developed country like the US spends around 2.8 trillion dollars on healthcare which means that every sixth dollar is spent on healthcare. This amount alone would become the fifth largest economy of the world after US, China, Japan and Germany. If that was not enough, the US government loses US$260 billion annually by not taxing health insurance benefits. The United States spends three times as much on hospital administrative costs than on all professional sports combined.

In comparision, things in India are very different, The World Health Organization's 2000 World Health Report ranked India's healthcare system at 112 out of 190 countries.

The Indian healthcare annual spend is US$100 billion which is almost equivalent to US$100 per person per year as against US$7285 in USA and a global average of US$802.The healthcare spend when compared on the basis of public-private contribution depicts a skewed picture in India where ~75% of the spend is by the private sector, whose primary goal is to make money. The growth in the Indian healthcare sector is poised to be one of the largest in the world. It's expected to grow to 280 billion by 2020 – a compounded annual growth rate of 22%. Since out of pocket spend is high, we are caught in this vicious web of profitability being at the core of quality healthcare.

- Indians spend an average of 58% of their total annual expenditure when hospitalised.
- Over 40% of Indians borrow heavily or sell assets to cover expenses.
- Over 25% of hospitalised Indians fall below poverty line due to hospital expenses.

"[11]Most of the debate around healthcare touches upon the overall spends and the allocations that follow. Actually some of the worst form of excesses, misappropriations and mismanagement happens under the broad head of

health spend in India, as SPR Foundation (IndiaSpend) has repeatedly found."

"Corruption in India's health sector: Begin with the reform of medical education"

An article by Radha Viswanathan highlights the core of this issue. She cites the example of Dr. David Berger, a public health specialists who came to India and worked as a volunteer in a charitable hospital in North India. Dr. David wrote an essay which was published in British Medical Journal dated May, 2014. The essay was titled corruption ruins the doctor-patient relationship in India and focusses how the public and private healthcare in India is rotting and needs an immediate intervention from agencies – both national and international. She emphatically states that "[12]At the lowest rung of this monumental ladder of corruption is the system of admissions to the private medical colleges that currently train doctors in 190 out of 350 medical colleges all over India. The 'capitation' fee or bribe as a precondition for admission is an astronomical sum which far exceeds the earning capacity of fresh passouts from such colleges. The quest for 'return on investment' in medical education begins early and serves as a strong disincentive to fresh graduate doctors working as generalists in rural areas, and paves the way for the practice of "medicine for maximum profit" in urban areas. The acute shortage of institutions that produce health workers at all levels – doctors, post-graduates, nurses, para-medics, community health workers – puts an unnecessary premium on the seats, setting in motion the vicious cycle of corruption"

Fact # 5 Iatrogenic Diseases – a silent killer

"[13]unlike pilots, doctors don't go down with their planes.", Dr Joseph Britto stated in an article in New York Times.

Dr Britto is a former intensive care doctor.

According to a report published in 2013 in National Centre of Policy Analysis,

"[14]An estimated 10 percent to 20 percent of cases are misdiagnosed, which exceeds drug errors and surgery on the wrong patient or body part, both of which receive considerably more attention."

Each year patients in hospitals get more than 1 million infections. A Harvard study of six hospitals showed that there are 20 percent chances of being harmed if you checked in there. Healthcare facilities are only 50 per cent compliant with hand washing. Stethoscopes carry bacteria like staph and yet, 50 per cent of doctors have never disinfected their stethoscope!

"[15]Nearly Nine Million (8,925,033) people were hospitalised unnecessarily in 2001. In a study of inappropriate hospitalisation, two doctors reviewed 1,132 medical records. They concluded that 23 per cent of all admissions were inappropriate and an additional 17 per cent could have been handled in outpatient clinics. 34 percent of all hospital days were deemed inappropriate and could have been avoided. The rate of inappropriate hospital admissions in 1990 was 23.5 per cent."

In most of the cases, an invasive and radical method like surgery is not the only option left. Most of the times there are alternate paths which can be followed, but as Dr Ido Weinberg has said and I quoted him before too, the decision of a doctor is influenced by multiple factors which might not be in alignment with a patient's best interest. Here is some data which might open your eyes:

"[16]In 1974, 2.4 million unnecessary surgeries were performed, resulting in 11,900 deaths at a cost of US $3.9 billion. In 2001, 7.5 million unnecessary surgical procedures were performed, resulting in 37,136 deaths at a cost of US$122 billion (using 1974 dollars)."

[17]Approximate deaths per year:

- 12,000 – unnecessary surgery
- 7,000 – medication errors in hospitals
- 20,000 – other errors in hospitals
- 80,000 – infections in hospitals
- 106,000 – non-error, negative effects of drugs

Everyone is out there to make money from your sickness. Hospitals, insurance companies and other institutions have their representatives, but who represents you? Who is your medical advocate? If all this scientific knowledge have such short shelf-lives, what is that knowledge that is eternal? What is your role in this entire scenario or drama triangle? Are you the victim, hero or the villain? Are you God or the disciple with blind faith?

FOUR

MD: Medical Deity

There's a commonly heard joke that the MD, after a physician's name, stands for "Medical Deity". But when exactly did this phenomenon come into play during the evolution of medicine? It certainly was not ceremonial. It happened gradually and became a social construct over time. This construct is now so deeply-rooted that many doctors unknowingly started believing that they are supreme. The notion of doctors as being God-like has its roots in patient expectations and the transference of power and control, from patient to physician.

The practice of medicine has traditionally been viewed as a noble profession that brings new life into the world, saves lives and becomes the benefactor of hope for those who are sick and distraught. It is easy to see how these actions can bestow an almost magical quality on the doctor. Physicians, in turn, have internalised many of the qualities that are necessary for them to fulfill these lofty expectations. According to the noted US physician, Dr Lewis Thomas, (*The Youngest Science*[1] *1995 Edition*),

> *"Self-confidence is by general consent one of the essentials of the practice of medicine, for it breeds confidence, faith, and hope."*

Dr Nassir Ghaemi[2], Director of the Mood Disorder Programme at Tufts Medical Center in Boston, quotes in his article in *Psychology Today*"[3]The concept of medical godhead reflects a mistaken notion of medicine, in my view; I call it Galenic, because it stems from the medical theory of Galen (Greek physician, surgeon and philosopher in the Roman empire), which has seeped into our profession and our culture after two millennia of wide acceptance. This is the view that nature causes disease, and that the doctor fights nature to cure the disease. The doctor provides the cure: only a step is left to godhead."

Interestingly, Dr Nassir further discusses that he believes that every doctor is aware that he is not God; yet at some level, is disappointed by that fact. Nassir believes doctors would not mind being thought of as gods, if it were possible, and patients accepting their divinity.

"But it does not work that way. Psychoanalysts have a concept for all this; they call it 'transference'. The idea is that patients transfer feelings, from somewhere other than the real doctor-patient relationship, to their doctors. The doctor is overvalued, and becomes a god, or demeaned, and viewed as lower than swine. Often, the one precedes the other. Neither is true.

Like the Greek divinities, doctors who play God, or who are seen as Gods, are seen to suffer one prime weakness: hubris. Doctors are arrogant; perhaps they are entitled, if in their expertise, they excel; yet arrogance is arrogance, and it feels distasteful. Arrogance is an odd thing, though, for, as Benjamin Franklin described, one could even have pride in not being prideful. It is hard to be truly and knowingly humble."

"Flattery corrupts both the receiver and the giver."
– Edmund Burke

In a desperate attempt to rely on someone else completely to get cured, patients give disproportionate value to doctors, which eventually resulted in something that we know as The God Complex! As sighted in Diagnostic and Statistical Manual – IV[4],

"God Complex is a pervasive pattern of grandiosity (in fantasy or behaviour), need for admiration, and lack of empathy."

Further, the Segen's Medical Dictionary defines it as a popular term for a personality flaw, commonly seen in physicians, especially surgeons, who perceive themselves as omniscient – i.e., God-like – and thus, treat others as mere mortals.

The problem is that medicine is not a science; it is an art, as William Osler said, based on science. As with any art – and even with science – there will be error.

An article titled *Professionalism and the God Syndrome*[5] published by Harvard Crimson in 1973, explains this in the American context:

"The contemporary physician is not a divinely-endowed medicine man, and yet society has dictated that he should have God-like attributes. Although he is actually a craftsman, many would deny him the human right to be fallible. He is not supra-human, but rather he is subject to the same fallibility as his human peers. The contemporary American physician enjoys an inflated aura of ultra-professionalism, one not so readily attainable by any other occupational group in our society. Indubitably this in itself has become a source of contention between the doctor and his patient, paternalism being the most definable of the malignant outgrowths.

Clearly the physician cannot have the upper-hand in decision-making. We must view him as a craftsman with indispensable technical expertise, but we cannot allow him to assume the position of a God."

"To Err is Human." – Alexander Pope

More often than not, we come across physicians who feel they can never be wrong. The reason for such a flawed belief can be their successful careers. But may I pose one simple question here? What is the definition of their success? Is removing a breast skillfully without any complications on the operation table called success? What if that breast never required removal in the first place?

One of our TMC members is a 63-year-old lady who was diagnosed with breast cancer (Infiltrating Ductal Carcinoma). She belonged to a family which is amongst the oldest established business houses in the city, with a very strong global and social network.

But like everyone does, they asked someone in the family for advice. This family doctor was an onco-surgeon and they felt blessed that he was going to be the treating physician as well. The family panicked and complied with the family doctor's advice to operate immediately. In normal practice, it is the tumour type that decides the treatment path and whether an oncosurgeon, medical oncologist, radiation oncologist and a palliative physician must get involved, and at what point. But so blind was their faith, that they did not involve anyone else at the first stage. They didn't even explore their options, despite being in a city like New Delhi where there are multiple JCI accredited hospitals and internationally-acclaimed doctors.

They eventually got her operated at a local hospital by this relatively less-experienced onco-surgeon, just based on family relations and trust. The next course of action recommended by this surgeon was chemotherapy and hormone therapy. Now, this was not his domain, so he referred them to another specialist from their religious community who was a medical oncologist. This oncologist wanted to start chemotherapy yesterday, forget even waiting for a week or a month.

The family again went into a tailspin and consulted eight different specialists. Six out of eight doctors insisted on starting chemotherapy and were deciding on the cocktail of drugs to prescribe.

The patient opposed chemotherapy and the family wanted a doctor to take that decision on her behalf, so they contacted Texas Medical Concierge. We started by consulting a local medical oncology specialist – Dr Rakesh Chopra and another, Dr Suresh Advani in Mumbai. Both of them were nowhere near as brutal; they wanted to wait and probe further and felt there was no sense of urgency as such. Rather, the urgency was being created artificially.

These two doctors were far more experienced than the rest and were open to discussions and global expertise. In this case, TMC further consulted Dr Matthew Ellis, director of the Breast Cancer Unit at Baylor St Luke's, leading hospital at the Texas Medical Center. He opined that for such cases, radiation was the first line of treatment, and removing the breast was completely unnecessary. If at all a partial lumpectomy would have sufficed.

Unfortunately in India, there is a tendency to go for more radical surgeries with complete disregard for the cosmetic or emotional impact of the treatment.

This global expert, during the consult, evaluated the benefits of chemotherapy by evaluating the lady in totality, and came to the conclusion that there was not going to be a more than a five percent advantage of this aggressive treatment over hormone therapy alone.

The lady had many comorbid conditions like hypothyroidism, diabetes mellitus and coronary artery disease, and by now, she was also clinically depressed. He considered her as a human being with cancer and not just a localised mass of disease. Under the circumstances, keeping in mind the patient's unwillingness for chemotherapy, he advised 10 years of hormone therapy as standalone treatment. As for the family surgeon afflicted with God complex, he too was invited to be a part of this tele-medicine consult. And what surprised me the most was that a moment before entering the video conferencing room, he had vehemently said – the next course of action was a chemotherapy drug called Paclitaxel and there was no other choice. After the meeting, he changed his stand and denied that he had ever suggested chemotherapy!

Is this called success?

Sadly, I learnt it the hard way. At every turn of my life in the medical industry, I noticed that such practices were indirectly harming more than healing. In our concierge medicine practice, we constantly have to battle inflated egos of doctors when we request them to be a part of second opinion consults with another specialist. They blatantly tell us that they have given their opinion and that's it. As if their word is law! There is very little openness to collaboration or reasonable doubt.

Patients in our part of the world tend to get treated by the first specialist they visit. In USA, things are a little different because of their sue-happy citizens. Did you know that in the United States, 15 million civil cases are filed annually[7]? Hence, there is more accountability and specialists welcome second opinions since malpractice laws are very stringent.

"[6]But decisions associated with medical issues are often complex, thanks to numerous unknowns and the uniqueness of each person's body" – as discussed extensively in Jerome Groopman and Pamela Hartzband's book, *Your Medical Mind.* According to them, most of us believe we are rational decision makers.

In a review by Dr Daniel J in the NY times, he comments on the book saying,

"[7]Suppose you've just found out that you or a loved one has prostate cancer. Nearly every urologist would recommend radical surgery to remove the organ. Sounds reasonable, doesn't it?"

They look at the numbers more closely. "Prostate cancer is slow-moving; more people die with it than from it. According to one 2004 study, for every 48 prostate surgeries performed, only one patient benefits – the other 47 patients would have lived just as long without surgery. Moreover, the 47 who didn't need the surgery are often left with an array of unpleasant and irreversible side effects, including incontinence, impotence and loss of sexual desire. The likelihood of one of these side effects is over 50 percent – 24 of our 47 will have at least one. This means a patient is 24 times more likely to experience the side effect than the cure."

"The focussing illusion", they write, "neglects our extraordinary capacity to adapt, to enjoy life with less than 'perfect' health."

The issues of God complex are universal and the Internet is filled with forums where patients express their frustration. The following excerpt makes an interesting read.

"[8]I've always wondered why surgeons seem to be more affected by the famous God complex that seems so prevalent in the medical profession. Recently, my cousin brother underwent surgery, as I talked about in my previous post, and the surgeon, who operated on him, whilst perfectly competent, also demonstrated this uppity demeanour. She strode into the OT (fashionably late) without seeing him pre-op, and didn't even check on him post-op. During the surgery, she didn't bother to reassure him; it was the nurses who did this. Now don't get me wrong, I'm not slagging surgeons. I know many fantastic surgeons, and hope to be one myself someday. I just think they could tone down their ego sometimes.

Not all ego is bad; I'm a Donald Trump fan and he's known for espousing the belief that a healthy ego leads to a higher quality of work. And this is true as long as it drives surgeons (and indeed any other worker) to perform better, but it's completely unnecessary when it causes them to ignore patients, shout at nurses and look down on doctors from non-surgical specialties. And abuse medical patients. Especially when they abuse medical patients. But that's an embarrassing story best saved for another day." – Anonymous Blogger.

"[9]I have only ever met two doctors that I liked. I liked them because they treated their patients like they were human, with respect and dignity. I can't stand the God complex that almost all of them get. I hate how they almost always disregard the mental/emotional aspect of people. It's like every patient is just a body. I believe that every doctor

should have a major bone broken, major surgery, and spend at least a week laid up in the hospital. That way they can understand how these things affect you on a personal level and not just a physical one. I have come to detest the way that a lot of doctors think that they are in total control and nothing matters, but what they think and want. They have lost sight of the fact that the patient decides what they do and not them. If the patient doesn't want something done it doesn't get done, no matter what the doctor thinks." – Anonymous Blogger.

Here is another interesting experience of a medical student in the doctors' defense, she says:

"[10]*I have been working in the medical field for five years now, and I can tell you at first, many doctors seem like pricks. Although it is true that many physicians forget that their name is followed by M.D. and not G.O.D., the more you are exposed to medicine, the more realistic your perceptions become. After I began working with doctors, I changed my major at the university to pre-nursing because I thought that would be the only way to really take care of people and keep personable and grounded. After continued exposure, I realised that the doctors that are good are REALLY good and I went back on the pre-med track and haven't looked back since. The doctors that often come off with this attitude, at least in my experience, are cardiothoracic surgeons, trauma surgeons and interventional cardiologists. These guys also by far have one of the highest stress environments when it comes to critical patients. Literally, every second counts and minor discrepancies can lead to the permanent injury/death of the patient for which they will be held responsible. Therefore, these guys tend to be the pickiest, crankiest and most demanding, but for good reason."* – Anonymous Medical Student

For sure, the relation between the doctor and the patient has frayed in the last few decades, and extensive research and specialisation has made it more complex. Technology and the revival of faith in ancient systems of medicine based on holistic health and another dimension, adds to this complexity. Textbooks and classroom education with clinical training might not be enough. We need a new perspective altogether.

"The cure of the part should not be attempted without the cure of the whole." – Plato

In the medical profession, specialists elicit respect and high esteem from people from all walks of life. Super specialisation is so advanced that it is not only based on organ systems but is disease based. There are several sub specialisations under ophthalmology for instance, like – cornea and external disease, neuro-ophthalmology, pediatric ophthalmology, ophthalmic pathology, ophthalmic plastic surgery, glaucoma, vitereoretinal diseases.

However, Gestalt psychology believes that medicine is not mathematics. It is not necessary that the characteristic of the sum of parts would be the same as the characteristic of the whole. The whole exists independently and is entitled to have its own nature, reaction and metabolism. Physicians often tend to get so consumed in their branch of medicine that they miss connecting the dots.

Another member of our TMC concierge programme was a little child. When he was three years old, he woke up one morning with a droopy eye. The parents rushed to the best eye specialist in New Delhi – someone who had sophisticated bedside manners and who spent a lot of time discussing various subjects like social trends, photography etc. He is usually very open to questions and is accessible; hence easy to trust. This brilliant doctor prescribed eye drops and treated the little boy for almost a month. He didn't find it important enough to evaluate the child and not just his eye. The child's condition did not improve and one fateful morning he experienced a seizure. The family eventually found out that the underlying cause of the drooping eye was neurocysticercosis, a tapeworm in the brain. Specialists have a tendency to focus on their organ of expertise and on symptomatic relief.

Typically, a specialist goes through nine years of education, making him/her develop a tunnel vision. But every physician inherently is aware of his or her limitations. Then why not be open about those limitations and take some action? Why not focus on healing and not treating? Their egos prevent them from collaborating to overcome this very natural occupational hazard. This is often because they are possessive and territorial about their patients and they don't want to lose them to someone else.

Without the correct application of a collaborative scientific process, there can be no advancement of knowledge. Open debate and discussion should be encouraged, not suppression or dismissal of evidence that does not support a particular theory.

In our private health management practice, our medical team collectively views each of our members as a whole person. We evaluate each case from nine perspectives so that we look at a problem from different lenses. Our job is to then refer them to the best disease-based specialist and then integrate those specialists to work in a complementary fashion. As a result, a lot of our clients end up consulting yoga, naturopathy or other ancient medicine specialists.

Not once has it happened that the treating modern medicine specialist has agreed to be a part of this alternative medicine consult. The oncologist feels degraded if we ask him to be part of the Ayurvedic consult. They are not willing to work as a team and integrate their approaches. Each approach has its area of impact and drawbacks.

However, not all physicians are like this. They do collaborate within their team and departments. Hospitals have tumour boards where supposedly each case is discussed as a group. Specialists do refer cases all the time but they do so either because they know the problem is clearly not their specialisation or because they have done what they could and can't do more to provide relief or a *cure*. In our experience, they tend to refer cases to known doctors within their network and not necessarily a global authority on that particular disease or set of problems.

Very rarely do they refer because they want another expert's view for confirming their diagnosis or line of treatment. I can literally think of a handful of Indian doctors who are willing to collaborate with a multi-disciplinary team. In my experience, almost invariably, the physicians who are open-minded are actually the ones who have the patients' best interest in mind. For them, they are not focussed on getting that intellectual high from "see I was right" or "I told you so".

But let's not blame it on these poor helpless doctors who are a part of something larger – a capitalist world where their livelihood depends upon the income they generate. Many have targets to meet and corporate directives to comply with. There are many vested interests at play; the system is often dysfunctional and blame cannot be simply imposed on just physicians and clinicians. There are other stakeholders like policy makers, researcher firms, public health practitioners, pharmaceutical companies and patient groups, who are equally responsible.

"The good physician treats the disease; the great physician treats the patient who has the disease."
– William Osler

While the God complex has been noticed and the frustration of patients has been registered all across the world, both patients and future doctors are being nurtured to escape the infliction of God complex.

Medical schools globally are starting to train doctors in softer skills and grooming them to be more amiable and less intimidating to patients. Further, patients are getting smarter and better informed, so less intimidated by doctors in turn. However, we haven't completely gotten away from the syndrome so perfectly described by Alec Baldwin's arrogant surgeon in the movie "Malice":

> *"[11]When someone goes into that chapel and they fall on their knees and they pray to God that their wife doesn't miscarry or that their daughter doesn't bleed to death or that their mother doesn't suffer acute neural trauma from postoperative shock, who do you think they're praying to? ... You ask me if I have a God complex. Let me tell you something: I am God."*

But there have been baby steps away from the omniscient doctor. The Federal Agency for Healthcare Research and Quality in Washington has begun a new campaign to encourage patients to ask more pertinent questions and to prod doctors to elicit more relevant answers. Patients are often scared to ask questions and are often incompetent medically to represent themselves in front of their doctors. They tend to think, "He's a doctor. He knows the best. Who am I to ask a question?"

Dr Groopman talks about this change in his book *How Doctors think*, and a book review published in New York times[11] by Michael Crichton takes the idea further:

"[12]In recent years, there has been a sharp reaction against the 'catch as catch can' approach to teaching diagnosis that prevailed when he was in medical school, where trainees would watch senior doctors and somehow absorb their way of thinking. But he is critical of much of the thinking, now in vogue. Today's physicians are increasingly encouraged to behave as if they were computers, and to reason from flowcharts and algorithms. This is intended to produce better diagnoses and fewer errors; it is also embraced by insurance companies, who use it to decide which tests and treatments to approve. This approach can be useful for *run-of-the-mill* diagnosis and treatment – distinguishing strep throat from viral pharyngitis, for example. But for difficult cases, he finds it limiting and dehumanising. He is similarly critical of generic profiles, classification schemes that draw statistical portraits of disease states. They encourage the doctor to focus on the disease, not the patient, and so may lead him to miss the particular manifestation in the particular sufferer."

I find it fascinating to view this discussion against the backdrop of the evolution of medicine and appreciate the way Dr Nassir has emphatically summarised it in his writings:

"[13]The other view, long lost but deeply correct, I think, is the Hippocratic view of medicine: The idea here is that nature heals disease, as well as causes it, and the role of the doctor is to help nature in the healing process. The doctor is the not the central hero, but the handmaiden to nature. This does not mean that cure does not occur, but it occurs less than we think, and nature deserves the credit, not any human being. There is no room for doctor as God, and our purposes are more humble: to cure sometimes, to heal often, to console always.

Medicine is a complex affair; we frequently do not do

justice to what our patients suffer and what they need. Pretending to know more than we do only makes matters worse. But being honest about what we do *not* know is not a sign of weakness."

Many patients express disgust on several forums making such strong remarks as below:

"[14]The intellectual gifts and volumes of integrated knowledge that a doctor must possess should be implemented with humility and a heart to serve people with your abilities. Someday those uber-arrogant surgeons may find themselves in a state of sickness or physical disrepair, and the perspective will come around.

Doctors bleed, breathe, and are subject to time and illness just like everyone else. It's all well and good to take pride in your work and accomplishments, but to serve all patients with humility and compassion reveals a sterling character."

Finally, how many doctors truly abide by the Hippocratic Oath which clearly says that:

> *"[15]I will use treatments for the benefit of the ill in accordance with my ability and my judgment, but from what is to their harm and injustice I will keep them."*

This awareness of their ability is the key and stepping up to take responsibility of keeping the patient from harm – whether it be the harm of their arrogance, their lack of empathy or their God complex is also equally vital.

I cannot simplify this further as it is done through a beautifully woven web of words in a poem called *Doctors* by Anne Sexton, who eventually committed suicide.

Doctors

They work with herbs
and penicillin
They work with gentleness
and the scalpel.
They dig out the cancer,
close an incision
and say a prayer
to the poverty of the skin.
They are not Gods
though they would like to be;
they are only a human
trying to fix up a human.
Many humans die.
They die like the tender,
palpitating berries
in November.
But all along the doctors remember:
First do no harm.
They would kiss if it would heal.
It would not heal.
If the doctors cure
then the sun sees it.
If the doctors kill
then the earth hides it.
The doctors should fear arrogance
more than cardiac arrest.
If they are too proud,
and some are,
then they leave home on horseback
but God returns them on foot.

FIVE

Life is by Choice not by Chance

Our body is not an independent entity; it's a reflection of the choices we have made. It's a reflection of our duties, our relationships, and our possessions. We are so focussed on the outside that when we neglect our body, we neglect our mind and we neglect our spirit.

My doctor failed to be my God when I realised he fails to see me as a whole person with dreams, aspirations, anger and life circumstances.

For him, I was merely a body infected with disease. But I was and I am more than a combination of organs working in synchrony.

Ardently following Dr Gershom Zajicek's work, I strongly agree with him that a different approach has to be taken and the entire problem has to be considered with a new perspective. Metaphysics in medicine is one such approach which can perhaps answer this question. The modern medicine sees health and disease merely as a relationship between host and the parasite and hence fails. Metaphysics adopts a more coherent philosophy and tries to address the complex dynamics of mind-body relationships, healing and illness.

I understood this through a very personal experience that tormented me for over two years, eventually leading to the wisdom I have now acquired.

> *"Healing is a matter of time, but is also a matter of opportunity."* – Hippocrates

JUNE 2010, LONDON

We are spending time with some close business associates and enjoying exquisitely crafted Scandinavian food at a Michelin star restaurant, Texture, in Portman square. We come back and I feel a small itchy rash behind my knees. I ignore it and go to sleep. The next day was the day Karan and I had been dreaming of for a long time. We were going to sign a deal on a flat that was breathtakingly beautiful facing Hyde Park. However, we decided against it after an emotionally draining and dramatic family meeting with my mother-in-law.

Our elder son Aaryaman aged 10 at the time was studying at Ludgrove, an English preparatory school which is over 200 years old. My son needed me, so I started finding reasons to be in London ranging from an MBA to expanding the family business.

The rashes were increasing, but I was too distracted by the preparations for the aristocratic champagne picnic basket I had to prepare for the school's annual sports day.

It was a fanfare where parents displayed their vintage cars, wealth and style. Everything was perfect – from fine food to fine people and fine crockery. Throughout the day I felt great but at night I felt the itchy rash again. Only this time I could see bumps appear on my legs. I thought it was an allergy and popped an Allegra. The rash would come and go but the issue was steadily getting worse.

We came back to India and the rash turned into full blown hives. It would come every single night. The wheals were massive bumps that would cover my entire body. They hurt and they itched! I went to see a leading so-called celebrity dermatologist in New Delhi and she casually said,

> *"There is no reason for this, you should take three antihistamines a day and that's it."*

That's it? Is this the way I was supposed to live for the rest of my life?

I was so miserable that I took the pills diligently. In fact, I would have done anything else she would have told me to. I was so drugged with these pills but my superwoman syndrome and miss do-it-all attitude got me by. I fought all the dizziness and continued to focus on my GMAT and my start-up with my business partner Becky. Things were not improving, in spite of the doctor changing the drug combination several times. In fact, it got worse! I started waking up to a randomly swollen eye or a lip to which my son Ashvath would joke,

"Mom you have a half Angelina Jolie lip."

One day the swelling appeared in my throat and I could not breathe. The lips were swollen, way beyond any sexy Angelina Jolie look. Karan rushed me to the hospital where they jabbed me with steroids and intravenous antihistamines. I decided to change my dermatologist and saw someone else the very next day. She told me that she wanted to know the cause behind my Urticaria and that I must do an allergy test. So I have these tiny needles stamped into my arms with over 60 different allergens.

It comes out that I am allergic to almost everything – grass, dust and dogs, including foods I consume on an hourly basis – pepper, lentils, papaya, banana, peanuts, potatoes, and hence vodka. That explained why the hives went berserk in Russia the previous month. Well, to cut the long story short, she changed my anti-allergy medicines and things were a little better. But not a single night had passed when I did not have wheals. The dermatologist then asked me to inject my body with a special concoction which was basically measured doses of the things I am allergic to so that I build immunity towards my allergens.

This was totally not sustainable, so life carried on in misery for two years now. One day Eva, my soul sister, friend and philosopher met me while waiting to pick up our kids at the American Embassy school. She asked me how I was and I said my allergies were killing me. She fleetingly told me in her Spanish accent

"Anchaal you are a psychologist! It's all in your mind!"

This was a passing remark but it set me thinking and I started researching old journals books and the Internet. There were very few studies that could give me an answer until I read a paper titled *Studies of the Personality of Patients Suffering from Urticaria* by E. D. Wittkower (MD).

Here, he cites the case of a physician who since childhood had been able to produce urticarial wheals on demand on his arms and legs and another patient who could produce it on an exact spot on his forehead. They also established that 35 percent of the cases in their study spontaneously stated that they missed parental affection especially maternal affection as children. In 19 out of the 25 patients studied, disturbing events of the nature described preceded the onset of their urticaria.

Research concluded that nobody would deny or dispute the importance of an allergy, but the view seems to be justified, "*that the immunobiologic approach does not give the final and only answer to the question of the etiology of urticaria and allied disorders. The interrelationships between allergic and emotional factors have been discussed elsewhere in several other researches.*"

Evidence obtained regarding the personality of patients suffering from urticaria suggests that urticaria is a disease which occurs in individuals who have been or have felt chronically deprived of affection. Who have always longed for it and felt frustrated because their basic need was not gratified. It has been shown that situations which objectively or subjectively intensified either their need for affection or their sense of frustration precipitated the onset or recurrence of urticaria.

This study was an eye-opener for me. I knew there was an underlying psychological cause. However, it was only five months later that I solved the mystery. Karan and I were at the Copacabana Palace Hotel in Rio De Janeiro. I told Karan that I think my urticaria is gone and I want to prove it to myself by eating this bowl of peanuts. Karan was furious at this childlike demand as we were in a Brazil on vacation and why would I want to screw things up and risk landing up in a hospital as a tourist. Stubborn as I am, I proceeded to eat my bowl of allergen and nothing happened! I had figured out the stressor.

It was a feeling and a longing that I had repressed into my subconscious. I was not aware that I yearned to have a home of my own that met my definition of beauty, luxury and comfort. I got married and moved into a home where my mother in-law was the lady of the house. In India we don't desert our parents by leaving the family home; the idea of a marriage is that two families marry not just two individuals.

Although it was a large home with lots of love and great food, it was an old home where three quarters of the property was not lived in. These portions had belonged to the extended family comprising of Karan's uncles, aunts and 15 cousins who had lived there many years ago. Although they moved out, we kept putting out the remodeling and built little sections on demand.

None of us wanted to bell the cat and take on a huge construction project in spite of desiring it. Just before the Brazil trip, I had taken a bold decision to start our construction because Aaryaman would go away to college in a couple of years from then, and this was not the childhood home I wanted him to have memories of. This home had no part of me in it. It was someone else's house I was living in.

One fine day, I requested my friend's mother if she could take on our project. Karan and mummy agreed, and they started breaking walls and drilling holes. My urticaria vanished the day the jack hammer came into our home and started tearing down the house a few days before our trip to Latin America for a conference in Buenos Aires, organised by Entrepreneurs Organisation. From that day till today, I have not had a single wheal! I realised on hindsight that my allergies started the very day my dream home in London, in spite of being so close to reality, became an unfulfilled dream.

Modern medicine is positioned towards curing diseases – that is, eliminating all evidences of disease. But does curing mean the same as healing? It does not, because healing involves becoming balanced and healing the person as a whole. It is hence important to challenge our current scientific mind and consider an alternative explanation at a metaphysical level.

STAGES OF DIS-EASE

I have a different perspective to disease which is based on my education as a clinical psychologist, ongoing study of the Vedanta Philosophy, and early exposure to spirituality.

My training in Cognitive Behavioral Therapy (CBT) which I used to treat people with a wide range of mental health problems influenced my personal school of thought. CBT is based on the idea that how we think (cognition), how we feel (emotion) and how we act (behaviour) all interact together. For me, I take the concept further, to state that feelings which we repress into our subconscious turn into disease.

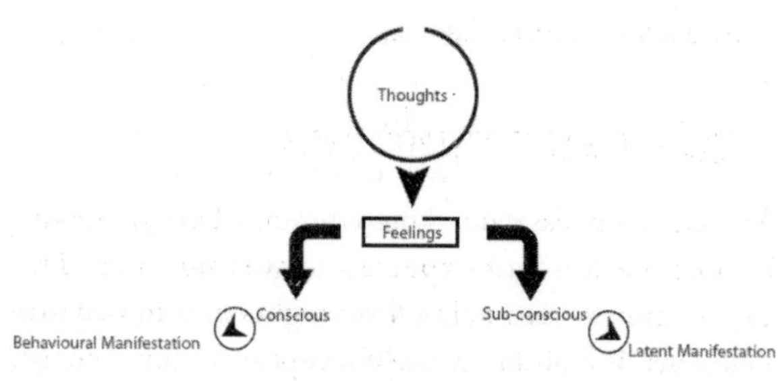

Illustration 2

Specifically, our thoughts determine our feelings and our behaviour. However, repressed feelings come out in the form of latent manifestations.

Possibly one of the most popular writer and philosopher who introduced metaphysics to lay people was Louise Hay. I am ever so grateful to her for sharpening my instincts and building on my academic knowledge. I strongly recommend every single person to read her book – *You can Heal your Life*. Much of what I am theorising below stems from her philosophy.

CBT on the other hand has its roots in the works of

behavioural scientists. In the 1960's, Aaron T. Beck, a psychiatrist, observed that during his analytical sessions, his patients tended to have an internal dialogue going on in their minds, almost as if they were talking to themselves.

I believe disease is a cry from your body, mind or soul, to look inwards and restore balance. We all have desires and expectations which are at the root cause of all discomfort, conflict and pain. Lack of control balance and awareness at a material, bodily, emotional, intellectual or spiritual level causes disease.

BLOCKAGES CAN BE AT DIFFERENT LEVELS

You are not at ease at a thought level, whereby creating a block because an expectation was not met. This expectation causes negative thoughts due to negative emotions. We all know the concept of positive energy and negative energy. An emotional blockage means that the negative energy has been trapped inside you. This accumulation of negative energy eventually manifests as a disease.

Types of desires or thoughts that cause these blockages could be either rational or irrational, and they can belong to the following realms:

Material Level – Material in this particular context means a need for temporary worldly objects which would eventually perish. For example, at a monetary level, we may be dissatisfied with the financial wealth we have. We feel lack of money for acquiring objects of desire.

Emotional Level – When our feelings are not reciprocated and our emotional desires are unfulfilled. For example, an emotional blockage can occur when we feel deprived of emotional needs like feeling frustrated, lack of emotional gratification or feeling oppressed as a victim of verbal abuse.

Physical Level – By physical, we are referring to thoughts and desires related to the body. Examples of such blockages are not feeling aligned with self-perception of beauty, a healthy body, being overweight or being underweight.

Intellectual Level – Intellect is developed over time with knowledge and experience and blockages at this level include disappointment with intellectual performance or arrogance at an intellectual level, an inability to agree with someone's school of thought, intolerance for others' religions, holding onto rigid ideology or feeling less knowledgeable than others.

Spiritual Level – Spirituality means being in synchrony with your deep conscious level. Spiritual blockage can occur when you are not being able to take responsibility for your own happiness and life and not feeling aligned to your core beliefs, deeper philosophy, belief system or values. For example, someone caught in a spiritual dilemma or someone who is forced to adopt a way of life contrary to his/her deeper philosophy.

Repressed thoughts and emotions manifest at different stages:

Stage 1 – Subtle Manifestation

Like the lid on a pot of boiling water trembles, there will be symptomatic release of the blockages through actions and happenings which may seem to be circumstantial or out of our control but the laws of nature, mentioned in our ancient scriptures, say otherwise. There are no accidents; everything that happens in our life occurs because we want it or have ordained it.

A subtle manifestation of a blockage can appear in one or more realms.

Material – Signs that there is some sort of blockage can manifest as minor irritants like theft, car breakdowns, or appliances, equipment and technology breakdowns.

Physical – You know you have some emotional blockages if you are neglecting or obsessing with your body. Blockages at a physical level may also be expressed through expressed through cravings, indulgent eating or drinking, smoking, addictions, laziness, procrastination or eating disorders.

Emotional – Unfulfilled desires and emotions can lead to emotional blockages which may be expressed through crying, screaming, criticising, fighting, blaming, phobias and so on.

Intellectual – A blockage may manifest itself at the intellectual level through seemingly less dysfunctional or rigid behaviours like fanatic or discriminatory actions or irregular behaviour at school or work, or working too hard or too little while acquiring intellectual knowledge or skills.

Spiritual – Constant confusion about the definition of spirituality, experimenting with different theologies, or rigidly following literal interpretations of religious texts.

Stage 2 – Gross Manifestation

If repressed issues are still not addressed or worked through, they lead to full-blown manifestations at either one or more levels.

Material – Unresolved blockages result in near fatal accidents, financial loss, change of home, loss of job, etc.

Physical – Due to lack of awareness and an inability to link the blockage to the behavior, your body and life starts to give you signals like aches, pain, sprains, minor injuries, inflammation, changes in weight, pimples, allergies, addictions, or constipation.

Emotional – An emotional breakdown can be in the form of a psychological or mental disorder. Further, Louise Hay and her disciples have provided a detailed list of metaphysical linkages of each part of the body to the plausible emotional blockage. For example, the liver represents repressed anger, and lungs represent grief. I have compiled a very exhaustive list which I personally find useful for self-analysis. The list can be found in the last chapter.

Intellectual – Actions taken at an intellectual level that are self-destructive in nature, for example, poor decision-making or lack of judgment, clarity and focus.

Spiritual – Blockages at this level may lead to a quest for spiritual truth or blind faith in religious dogmas, gurus, astrologers, psychics, philosophies, abandonment of your inner journey, and so on. Spiritual blockages also create terrorism, riots, wars etc.

Stage 3 – Release of Blockages

Release of blockages through death depends on the nature of blockages we subconsciously or karmically check out. Death and the end of life stages are partial or indirect release of blockages when they become unmanageable and unbearable.

Material – Death through major expenditure on disease.

Emotional – Death through suffering and pain.

Physical – Death through physically degenerative and painful diseases.

Intellectual – Death after prolonged illnesses like Coma, Alzheimer's, Schizophrenia.

Spiritual – Death due to volunteer release

For those of you who find this concept very bizarre, this is another perception. We all have limited knowledge anyway.

By virtue of being human, we will all age and manifest disease at any of the stages above. Which stage a person might be in, at any given time depends on their level of awareness and inner control, how aware we are of who we really are, where we are at, how much resistance do we have, what our beliefs are, what we want and so and so forth.

You cannot correlate the severity of someone's blockage to the severity of their illness or condition. *You can't ever judge anyone's manifestation from the outside.* A conflict or an unresolved or unrecognised issue that might give your neighbor cancer might not even give you a pimple. It's very personal. It's called the journey of life and the beauty of nature is that no two lives are identical. Awareness at the levels above and trust in your own pure consciousness has to be a core belief.

Taking this thought a bit deeper, I believe that we may have a hidden reason for manifesting disease. In psychology, we term it as a *secondary gain.* Every manifestation is actually fulfilling your desire that you may or may not be aware of. The loss of holding on to the issue is perceived subconsciously as greater than its absence. For example, chronic pain or diabetes which may have no apparent cause, might be fulfilling some latent desire like the attention the patient gets from his or spouse. The need to deny the original cause of pain is intense, since that truth hurts more.

The bigger the blocked desire is, the more painful the manifestation will be. The longer the blockage is left unattended, the stronger the manifestation will be. I believe that our lives are a manifestation of our thoughts, feelings and actions.

The human body is a work of art and science made to perfection. Yet, most of us don't have faith in it and often we even view it as our enemy. While we do age with time, it's a battle that none of us can win.Your body doesn't need you to heal it. Our body's natural state is one of perfect health. Healing is not just about returning the body to that state of health. Healing is about unblocking what's in the body's way, in order to allow it to heal itself and return to its natural state.

While at no point do I suggest that modern medicine and its clinical approach be avoided in lieu of this approach, it is important to realize that symptomatic treatment and a clinical approach is equally important.

Most of us are aware that Steve Jobs regretted trying to cure his cancer with alternative medicine alone. He did not integrate technological advancements with his acupuncture sessions, naturopathy, spiritual and energy healing. As quoted by his biographer, "he regretted trying to beat cancer with alternate medicine for so long."

Blind faith and belief in the absence of scientific rigour is ignorance. I am a firm believer that cutting-edge technology and treatments must be deployed. We would be pre-historic if we decided to go back to herbs and witches. As per an article on the website of Indian Psychology Institute,

"[1]Scientists and spiritualists have been at opposite ends due to a fundamental theoretical problem. Therefore, is that whether a science originating from the mind can register, appreciate and study something beyond it?

In order to make a progress in both the disciplines one has to follow different and contradictory paths, which makes an interface difficult. The scientist must search for mind in the brain whereas the spiritualist strives to transcend both mind and brain."

As the Vedanta Philosopher Swamy A Parthasarthy vehemently reiterates, "The modern human intellect is blinded by ignorance. You must realise that you are born in captivity, you live in captivity and die in captivity. You are showed do's and don'ts, maxims and mandates by the world. Later in life, you are victimised by the community and the society you live in. As a result of these external pressures, your mind caves in. You remain enslaved to them."

Physicians in particular are forced to be such victims by virtue of their scientific and academic training. They feel compelled to disagree with these eternal truths which are nothing more than laws of nature.

SIX

Dear Doctor

In our minds, "doctor" as a word is opposite to the word "patient". This is just a construct that is psychologically established in our minds and it is hard to imagine a doctor as a patient. So much so that it's hard for doctors to accept themselves as patients.

"[1]As physicians, we are used to being the people in control in the healthcare setting. When the doctor becomes the patient, all perceived control is surrendered. No longer do we wear the magic white coat and wave healing hands over patients. Our daily intake and output is recorded. We are shipped all over the hospital for tests in unflattering, often risqué attire. Once the transition to patient is made, there is no going back. Nothing ever seems the same."

- Dr Kevin Campbell, MD, FACC[2], internationally recognised cardiologist

To become better doctors, doctors need to become better patients

It is believed that the journey from being a doctor to being a patient is a shocking transition. Being a patient should be a part of continuing medical training so that they can continue to get reality checks from time to time.

Research shows that doctors make very bad patients. They have high rates of mental health problems including anxiety, addictions and increased suicide rates. They are less likely to reach out for help, despite understanding their own condition and probably diagnosis too.

[3]A BMA survey of doctors found that over 50 per cent thought that their work had affected their health and over 30 percent dealt with this by self-prescribing. Less than 50 percent took sick leave and although most were registered with a GP (general practitioner), most consulted colleagues when ill, rather than seeing their GP. Doctors who tend to self-medicate, are reluctant to seek outside help or only do so at a late stage. Among their anxieties is often a fear of the stigma associated with illness.

Multiple reasons attribute to this occupational hazard that they face. There are also a number of myths associated amongst medical students which circle around doctors being mentally ill. They think that:[4]

- "If I have a mental health condition, it will damage my career prospects."

- "Staff will treat me differently if they know I have a mental health condition."
- "Seeking help is seen as a sign of weakness."

FIVE REASONS WHY DOCTORS MAKE BAD PATIENTS

1. Inseparable Professional and Personal Identity

> *"The surest way to corrupt a youth is to instruct him to hold in higher esteem those who think alike than those who think differently."*
> – Friedrich Nietzsche

The inception of being special starts right from the time when students enter medical school. Once they graduate, they get the tag of *doctor* which sticks to them not only in clinics but among friends, relatives and families too. While abandoning the medical self becomes a challenge, it diminishes their ability to seek help and there is a stigma associated with being ill. Their professional identity is almost inseparable from their personal identity. An article in *The Guardian* explains a doctor's fears about letting people know that he is sick:

"[5]I haven't told anybody at work. Why? I don't know, partly I see it as a sign of weakness. We are supposed to be curing people. We are not supposed to be weak. I don't want people thinking, 'He's gone bonkers.' And in the back of my mind, if something goes wrong, if I make a mistake, I don't want people thinking..." He trails off.

"It's a political business, being a hospital consultant. You don't show anybody any weakness. I don't want people thinking I need help."

2. Doctors are Busy Bees

"If you have no time to rest, it's exactly the right time"
– Mark Twain

Since many doctors work for almost 11 hours a day, it is extremely difficult for them to register with a general practitioner. Being a doctor, they are not able to take help during their work hours. Even after working for 11 hours a day or more, they realise that they are able to give little time to their patients.

Nancy Rappaport who is an assistant professor of Psychiatry at Harvard Medical School explains the need for doctors to give time to themselves. She says,

"[6]Giving of ourselves is essential to a doctor's work, but in many ways, realising our limitations and recognising our exhaustion is most important if we are to effectively take care of our patients and sustain our passion. It is when we neglect ourselves that potentially fatal errors can occur; asking for help and realising when we're over our heads are crucial to our performance and maintaining our humanity.

I've learned to recognise when it is critical to take care of myself, and I encourage all doctors to develop a pattern of self-care. It's necessary to prioritise time for family and for ourselves, allowing us to preserve our deep love for our healing craft, and the energy to keep doing it."

3. Inherent traits of a doctor's personality

Doctors are saviours and their entire training and professional life shapes the sub-strata of their minds, behaviours and personality, depending upon their circumstances and exposure. There are certain kinds of personality traits which act as a psychological barrier for reaching out for help[7].

Perfectionists ("I must do this right, mistakes are intolerable")
Narcissists ("I am the greatest")
Compulsives ("I must do this, and I can't give up till I finish")
Denigrators of vulnerability ("People who need help are failures. If I need help, I am a failure")
Martyrs ("I care for my patients more than myself, and my needs are secondary to those I treat")

4. Facing a Colleague as a Patient

There are many professional concerns stemming from the fear of illness that it may affect their careers. Many doctors find it embarrassing to visit a doctor who has been a colleague. This shift in power is unbearable for some of them. They are no more collaborating or referring or discussing a case. One of them is actually reaching out for help, which is rough on their ego.

Doctors report that if they are back to work after recovering from a certain ailment, there is a substantial lack of support from the colleagues. The colleagues, in turn, have an implicit belief that they are letting down the profession by being ill. Thus, there is a stigma attached with the label of any kind of medical condition for physicians.

5. They know too much

"Three-quarters of the sicknesses of intelligent people come from their intelligence. They need at least a doctor who can understand this sickness."
– Marcel Proust

As a patient, they are quick to pick up mistakes in their treatment, diagnosis or care; ironically, the same issues that they might have chosen to ignore while treating their own patients. Having a deep understanding of the medical condition often causes a conflict with the treating doctor or nurse as they try to take control of the situation.

"[8] The first or second time I saw a psychiatrist, I managed to pull the wool over their eyes – I'd done that through 10 years of therapy, too. It was not a normal patient-doctor relationship. I convinced the other doctor that nothing was wrong."

Knowing too much helps them deceit the other doctors due to which the situation can get worse.

Further, what complicates the whole scenario is that we are in the middle of a generational transition and it's imperative to ride this tide of inevitable change.

THE AGE OF MILLENNIAL PHYSICIANS

Gone are the days when the renaissance of technology had not touched our lives. Gone are the memories of having a family physician looking after you at home. Gone are the vivid visualisations of a village physician going door to door along with his compounder carrying the leather bag.

The bag that the compounder carried used to be a mini clinic packed with needles and glass syringes that needed boiling for sterilisation. It was a time when injections were supposed to be the remedy for all. The bottom part of the bag was full of medications contained in glass bottles, blood pressure cuff and other instruments which were used in rare cases. The bag defined the doctor.

So doctors carried vials of penicillin, adrenaline, coramine, theophylline,a box of Vitamin B12 capsules – the placebo that had always worked. Times have changed, and doctors today carry iPads and not bags. Every injection or pill they administer is heavily "Googled" by their patient, making it impossible to administer a placebo. The size of bulky instruments has shrunk to the arsenal that doctors carry with them and almost everything that is required can be kept in their white coat, which became a symbol of purity at the end of the 19th and the beginning of the 20th centuries. This is when medicine became the truly scientific enterprise we now know; the "whiteness" or "pureness" of medicine became reflected in the garb of physicians and, interestingly, nurses. Ironically, prior to white coats, they wore black uniforms signifying professionalism. Their clothes are changing and so are they.

PHYSICIANS BELONGING TO DIFFERENT GENERATIONS DIFFER IN TERMS OF CHARACTERISTICS

Characteristics that define and differentiate generations – while none of that data can paint a totally accurate picture of any one doctor, the research does allow us to cover the canvass in broad strokes. Robert Pearl who is the CEO of Permanente Medical group, states in his article in Forbes:

"[9]Baby Boomers (born 1946-1964) are known for their work ethic and long-term commitment to a single organisation. They've been willing to trade work-life balance for professional success,recognition and financial security.

Generation Xers (born 1965-1983) are comfortable moving between jobs and don't see themselves working for any one organisation their entire lives. They tend to prioritise a balanced lifestyle over financial gain.

Millennials (born 1984-present) expect to work with multiple employers and seek out cross-cultural and global opportunities. They too value flexibility in their work-life balance. They don't mind working hard but want to be judged on their output and results, not the total number of hours they put in.

And compared to their predecessor generations, millennials have a disproportionately stronger entrepreneurial spirit and prefer to work in efficient, fast-moving, team-based organisations.

Not all generational generalities are foolproof: Some baby boomer physicians are as high-tech as the savviest millennials and plenty of Generation X doctors put in long hours.

But on the whole, there are fundamental differences in doctors' work styles, communication habits and overall fondness for change in the context of a rapidly evolving health care world."

Millennials are taking over the world now. The future is all about them and how they approach healthcare and medicine. It is in doctors' hands that they decide to make a difference or not. But there are still some key points to remember. There is a need to alter the approach and see everything with a fresh perspective.

We faced the challenge that this issue posed in our practice. Our medical concierge team was once contacted by a lady in New York, extremely panicked that her daughter Olivia (name changed) had been in a road accident in a small town in the interiors of India. Immediately, we activated the air evacuation, but to the American family's horror, there are no Medivac helicopters in India. This family was an empowered family in every aspect – they had financial strength, education and a global network – hence, they had the right to demand quality and speed. Olivia was a true millenial, she knew her needs and was very aware of the treatment being administered to her. The next few days that followed were not just a patient's nightmare but a hospital's nightmare too. The doctors in India's premier medical hospital owned by a so-called celebrity doctor of the baby boomer generation, did not know what hit them.

They had no clue how to deal with an international family or how to meet global standards of care. Indian doctors would march into the room unannounced, with a halo around the senior-most doctor's head and an entourage of assistant doctors behind him, and rattle off instructions and options mechanically. Being a student of the alternative healing systems, Olivia was very sensitive to the energy of the people who entered her room, lying there with multiple fractures in her leg and severe pain which impacted her patience. The family would express their disgust and disappointment since they were empowered patients and not mere mortals at the mercy of these celebrated, worshipped physicians. The family was a family of lawyers. They respected physicians like any other professional who puts in years of hard work to get where they get.

As their concierge team, we were called in to co-ordinate all elements of care and to get them to New York for surgery as soon as possible, even if it meant chartering a 777 Jet that would fly nonstop. Olivia understood her medications, was medically very aware and knew everything. *Web MD* had to teach her about her situation. Indian doctors were not used to this; many see 50 patients a day who are uneducated, ignorant or servile. They did not pay heed to the fact that here was a family in shock, with absolutely no exposure to India, demanding that they be a partner in this entire escapade. This incident shook up the systems in the hospital and every single mistake was picked up; typically, the average patient would oversee it or be unaware of such issues. Mistakes the doctors made actually amounted to malpractice, but all these errors stemmed from the doctor's attitude and the arrogance of people on top who ran the facility.

Millennials do not accept the following attributes which these physicians presented:

1. **Poor bedside manners** – Walking in without introducing themselves, would not sit the family down and tell them in detail what their daughter's condition was, talking to the male member and ignoring the mother, not asking how they felt or what their needs were, lack of sympathy or empathy.
2. **Lack of coordination** – We would discuss the treatment in Olivia's room, keeping in mind her allergies, the hospital in New York's suggestions, and the treating doctor's opinion; the next thing we know is that the nurse had a different set of instructions. Had Oliva not checked each medicine they gave her, she would have not caught the nurse administering her medications that she was not supposed to have.
3. **Inflated egos beyond belief** – Being the best surgeons in their respective field by virtue of the number of surgeries performed, certainly is no reason for them to walk around as Demigods. This Ego translated into their behaviour and demeanour.
4. **Overseeing basic medical protocols** – Pain management, drug administration, and hand sterilising.
5. **Not up to speed with global healthcare trends** – Using barbaric tools, and not giving access to their medical records or to the patient the patient portal.

Here are some words of wisdom from some of the Texas Medical Concierge physicians who are young millennial doctors themselves. These concierge physicians not only have the medical training, but have been involved in interdisciplinary teams, been close with patients, and have presented cases to specialists around the world. Following are their recommendations for their colleagues, both young and old.

FIVE THINGS A MILLENNIAL DOCTOR OF GENERATION Y SHOULD DO TO RIDE THE TIDE OF CHANGE

1. Avoid the God complex

Dear doctor, please have an attitude of gratitude and feel thankful that you are in such a noble profession. Ego can consume you. It clouds your judgment and can influence your profession negatively. Accept responsibility for what you are capable of. Bad behaviour is a result of God complex and has a severe impact on you, your staff and your patients. The conflict between patients and nurses is also a common phenomenon, and between these battles of ego, it is the patient who is eventually victimised.

According to a special report published in 2009 about doctor-nurse behaviour survey,"[10]*While disruptive behaviour is terrible, no matter who the target is, the problem becomes especially worrisome when it affects innocent third parties – patients and their families. From making mean and insensitive comments within earshot, to behaviour that actually puts lives at risk, both physicians and nurses are guilty of putting patients in uncomfortable and downright dangerous situations."*

2. Refer, collaborate or let it go

It is obvious that you cannot be an expert in every single domain that medicine has. You are a human and it's okay if you are not sure about things. In every such case where you feel the case does not belong to you, do refer! The tunnel vision can be harmful for the patient and I know you have no intentions to hurt your patient. Refer it to the doctor whom you think is appropriate for the case. Don't refer it to someone because he or she is a good friend or a relative.

Collaboration is crucial. Ask for help, opinions and frame a decision while collaborating with other experts which might or might not be from modern medicine. Taking a second opinion does not mean that you lack skills or are under confident. It means that you are sensible and mature enough to understand the need of another perspective which can be beneficial for the case. The Medical Council of Ireland lists collaboration as one of the Eight Domains of Good Professional Practice.

"[11]Medical practitioners must co-operate with colleagues and work effectively with healthcare professionals from other disciplines and teams. He/she should ensure that there are clear lines of communication and systems of accountability in place among team members to protect patients."

Moreover, being inaccessible at times is completely understandable. In such situations, you can always nominate someone who has some idea about the patient and his/her medical history; and is qualified enough to explain medications, side effects and treatment protocols.

Intelligently, letting go is a skill that can be more helpful in increasing a doctor's business. Yes, you have a right to fire your patient. The Pareto Principle can be remembered here or as we know it – the 80/20 rule. It implies that 80 percent of your overall income is through 20 percent of patients or let's say 20 percent of time that you invest in good patients out of the entire lot.

And a higher percentage of time is being consumed by the other 80 percent of patients. So maybe, it is time to establish the balance, or maybe you can invest that time with your family?

3. Embrace technology or get left behind

Technology is your weapon. You are lucky to be born in an era when technology has metamorphosed everything, and the contribution of technology in the medical field is incredibly significant. Use it to your benefit. Dissolve the boundaries with an advanced communication. The whole world is at your disposal.

It is understandable that you can't help your patients with small little pieces of information they are curious about. There are more patients waiting for you to see them but if you don't have time to counsel or educate, then have a bank of resources or appoint someone from where the patient can get further answers.

Maintain your clients' data electronically for their sake and yours.

Digitise it and share the data that you are creating after examining the patient or after any other test, with them, so that it could be accessed by them and you whenever and wherever required. Disaster never comes knocking at your door announcing itself and in any such situation, this electronically recorded data would be immensely helpful.

4. Evaluate the patient as a whole

As narrated by a doctor himself,

"[12]To achieve care that truly addresses the whole person, behavioural and physical health care must be integrated. And they should be: Integration has been shown to improve health outcomes and reduce overall medical costs.

My tumour was completely removed, no further treatment was needed, and I have a good prognosis. For all this, I am grateful. But the outcome does not change what I found missing during my experience as a patient. Let's face it, caring for the entire individual – her head as well as her kidneys – is just good care. The kind we all want for ourselves and our families."

Just in case you are too busy, build up a good second line in command that does not miss the details. Never jump to conclusion in the absence of medical data or with partial information of symptoms. To make an intelligent and credible decision, you need information to analyse and evaluate. This information needs to be extracted from the medical history of the patient. If you are not accessible, delegate.

Happy patients are good patients. Being positive of a patient always helps himself and the doctor as well. The problematic patients would mostly be negative and would keep complaining and whining. They even might be abusive to you and your staff. Honestly, you really don't need that and it is your responsibility to stand for your staff. You can simply fire such patients.

5. Understand the Millennial patient

Millennials are emerging to be the top purchasers of all kinds of goods and services. But at the same time, they are smart, tech-savvy and conscious about everything. Doctors need to advance in their approach if they want to tackle the millennials.

According to an article[13] by Jess White who has been writing articles on health business for various publications, three ways that can help you deal with Millennials are:

Provide speedy healthcare

Millennials are fast and they want access to everything conveniently. They usually rely upon urgent care facilities and visit emergency rooms only when there is something very serious.

"[13]Millennials who do visit the hospital may need a bit more prompting to visit a primary-care doctor for regular follow-up appointments."

Stay connected

The Generation Y has grown up with the Internet. It feels natural for them to be connected through social media and it is likely that they will be checking the reviews of your medical healthcare services online.

More and more doctors use applications like Facetime, Whatsapp, Facebook and Skype.

"[13]It's also helpful for your hospital to have an active, positive presence on social networking sites. You may even want to hire a social media manager who can maintain your hospital's Facebook page while browsing sites like Yelp to check out how patients are rating your care."

Be cost conscious

Millennials are conscious about costs, probably more than the previous generations. They do think before spending and have several apps to run quick cost comparisons.

"[13]In fact, 41 percent of millennials surveyed said they'd only even consider receiving certain healthcare treatment after they've asked for and received an estimate of how much it'll cost them. And 54 per cent have actually delayed or avoided treatment because of cost."

As Louise Hay says, it important to do some mental house cleaning. Take a look at some of the beliefs that you may painfully have to get rid of – doctor and patient alike. "Every man is a divinity in disguise, a God playing the fool." – Ralph Waldo Emerson.

SEVEN

Patients – Judge Yourself

Everyone is vulnerable to sickness and disease. If doctors are not gods, you are not a superhero either. To think that sickness or accidents are meant for your neighbours and you are going to be an exception, is living in a fool's paradise.

If you are to be the CEO of your health, you need to shed your superhero cape and embark on a journey to discover the patterns of behaviours you use with regards to you or your family's healthcare.

In the previous chapter, we saw how doctors themselves make bad patients and that they need to step up the game to deal with the millennials. We as patients or as potential patients need to ensure that we are not dinosaurs either.

The world as we know it has changed tremendously since the advent of the Internet. With more choices at our disposal, there is more confusion and stress. Stress and lifestyle-related diseases are on the rise and the patient has Dr Google as their primary physician. These factors bring the onus of healthcare more on you than ever before. The old balance of power where the doctor had an authoritarian position has changed.

Healthcare today is different from yesteryears as it's characterised by the following factors:

- Doctor-patient relationship is more transactional
- Medicine is more super specialised and technology-based
- Primary care physician or family doctors are on the decline
- Person or family is responsible for all decision-making and healthcare coordination
- Medical data is stored in different places
- Diseases today are not caused largely by infections but by lifestyle choices

How a doctor treats you has a little more to do with you than you think. To be more in control of the equation between your physician and you, it's important for you to step up and take personal responsibility.

Live a life of choices and not chances – It all starts with a certain level of honesty. Establish consciousness and a connection with your body. Answer some hard-hitting questions like:

- Whose eyes do you view yourself from?
- Who do you compare yourself to?
- What is your definition of health?
- What illness troubles you the most?
- Which illness do you fear the most?

Try discussing such things with your family or friends, or journal it in your personal diary. This helps in reducing the emotional fluff around emotionally-laden words like cancer, paralysis, blindness and more. Now that your guards are down, please review the following information and try and take away what you can to be a conscious CEO of your health.

Rule # 1 – Prevention is better than cure

Do you have a medical insurance that covers all your needs and fears ? Have you heard of preventive medicine? Maybe you believe in the theory of karma and feel you have to passively accept what comes your way – whether it's the extra weight on your body or soaring insulin levels in your blood. It's your destiny, hence you are helpless. I urge you to probe further and truly evaluate or dig deeper into the philosophy of karma at the very least, to understand that it simply means that you get what you deserve based on your thoughts and actions. It's not about passive acceptance. Our body is our temple and it is our duty to have gratitude and respect for this marvelous gift of life that we have.

The first step is being smarter, organised and to value prevention. We all know a stitch in time saves nine. But I was surprised to learn that in India, almost 80 percent of cancers are diagnosed as late-stage cancers. Early detection of any disease betters your chances of cure. Day after day I am pained to meet clients who come to

TMC when all other roads are closed, and they just want to know their options now; or specialists refer them to us because they have done everything possible including several rounds of chemo, surgery and radiation; but there is no improvement.

The following case highlights an incomplete prevention strategy for 65 years old Mrs Khanna (name changed). She was a happy-go-lucky kind of person; loved to live a life of indulgence in food and friends. Typically, she saw a doctor only when she had an issue. She had some random preventive checkups done sporadically or under the instructions of her life insurance company.

In 2014, Mrs Khanna got some tests done, following which, reports were handed over to her. She read the reports in which it was written that X-ray findings were suggestive of Interstitial Lung Disease (ILD). Mrs Khanna probably skipped this detail or ignored it after reading, and continued her happy life since she felt no symptoms. A year later in 2015, she had a serious episode of breathlessness and the CT scan showed that 75 percent of her lungs were damaged. Since ILD is a progressive disease, the lung damage was irreversible. Imagine if we had caught it two years prior? Imagine if the family physician would have been a little more attentive and not so transactional? What if the radiologist who handed over the report told her in clear words that she needs to see a lung specialist?

This is not wishful thinking but it's actually called risk mitigation.

On the contrary, we also have young professionals who sign up for our concierge membership because they want someone to help them prevent getting sick. These are our ideal clients because they are pro-active, systematic and objective in their approach. They use our services to get all the medical intelligence, along with the concerned specialist who decides the next course of action. In our experience, millennials are getting a lot more progressive about taking charge of their health now than our parents or grandparents. The generation of baby boomers needs to catch up, as we are facing lifestyle and environmental pressures that create a need for us to be more proactive.

Rule # 2 – Don't be Reactive. Be Proactive

Pro-active people get things done, while reactive people have little control and are usually governed by external factors. How do you go about your healthcare in general? Do you go to a doctor when you are sick? Do you get preventive checkups done regularly? Or you just have a very casual and take-it-easy approach? Or worse, do you feel that if you don't know it, the problem does not exist and hence you can avoid a doctor completely?

If you are reading this book, you are likely to be educated, probably well-travelled, maybe even a doctor yourself. Nonetheless, you need to reflect and evaluate to understand if you have a casual approach to your health or your family's health. We need to consciously decide whether we want to spend time, money and energy on our health or disease – the choice is ultimately ours. Either way, it's hard work.

To prevent diseases, we need a sound mind and an able body which is nurtured. It requires a conscious effort to have a prevention plan drawn out by your family doctor, primary care physician, concierge physician or whoever else you entrust this job to. And yes doctors, you too need to appoint a CEO which cannot be you yourself, since you are attuned to a self-sacrificing nature.

Just like for our businesses, we have documented strategies; it important to have a written prevention strategy, which is addressing you as a whole. Having an incomplete or incompetent prevention strategy is equivalent to having none. If you are aware of business jargons, you may know the concept of SMART goals. Goals that are Specific, Measurable, Achievable, Realistic and Time-bound.

What's more surprising is when professionals, executives, business leaders or others with the means to shake a political party behave like blue-collar workers – forget even being managerial in their approach to healthcare.

One of our clients Mr Aggarwal (name changed) is a leading industrialist with a large family business of manufacturing. He came to us in a panic-stricken state, as he had been diagnosed with a tumour that was 5.8 * 10.4 * 16.3 cms in size, which is a size larger than a *tennis ball*.

At the age of 50, it was hard to believe how he could have been ignorant and casual about the pain in his back which radiated to his leg. The annual tests he underwent as preventive measure were not personalised to suit his symptoms. This tumour was estimated to be sitting there for a minimum of five years. We could have blamed it on a freak chance or lack of awareness, but what followed was a series of reactions that were chaotic. He was not clear in his mind and was now making wrong decisions at each step on his way.

Being in a joint family set up, there were too many bystanders – four brothers and their wives, a wife, two children and all the young nephews and nieces. In India it is common for the entire family to live together and the final decision is always taken by the eldest person in the house.

However in this case no one person was willing to step in and take control. They all started running from pillar to post trying to offer their two bits of a scatter-gun support. We got them a few domestic and global opinions which indicated the seriousness of his condition and the need to chart out a well-thought-out treatment regimen. The doctor who scared them the most and suggested to begin chemotherapy immediately was the one they believed, and the family blindly took the plunge. Chemotherapy is a very aggressive treatment where there are many factors that determine its efficacy. Couple of weeks later, the family again went into a frantic frenzy and began searching for global options; by now it was too late since they had started the chemo cycle. He was getting caught in a vicious cycle of reactive behaviours.

It's important to identify who is your family doctor or what they call in the US – a primary care physician (PCP). Hand him/her a list of expectations you have; find the job description that would help you outline the functions of a family doctor, appended at the end of the book.

In India, this concept has been lost. It was there in the past when family doctors made regular home visits and knew you as a whole human being. You may feel you have a family doctor, but ironically, if I call up your family doctor in India and ask them if they know your blood group, nine out of ten will say they don't. If they are the general managers of your health, have you empowered them? Do they have all your consolidated medical data available with them? How accessible are these physicians and this data? What is the network of this family physician? Are you aware of his/her strengths and limitations or do you just behave like a robot? You bet I have met many robots who in their professional lives are tyrants, but when it comes to blind faith in a family doctor, they become subservient and powerless.

Rule # 3 – Consolidate your medical records, prepare a brief clinical summary, and keep it accessible and up to date

Where is all your medical data? Is it scattered or all compiled and indexed? Is it in paper files or soft copies? Where is it stored? Who all know it's stored there?

Honestly, most people don't have satisfactory answers to these questions. On the contrary, we have clients who feel they are very well-networked into the medical fraternity. Since these people are influential, they can navigate their way by placing a phone call or two. Fortunately for them their children realise how limited this approach is and gift them a medical concierge membership to expand their options.

You won't believe how many calls we receive at TMC through the day asking for recommendations and priority appointments with celebrity doctors. As much as we would want to help them, we refrain from making any recommendations in the absence of a complete medical history. We do so because we believe that there are disease-based specialists, and finding the right doctor is imperative.

It's not possible to find the right doctor in the absence of a clear history or physician's evaluation. In all such cases, we either request them to go back to their family physician who knows them or come in along with their medical records for a two-hour long history session with our concierge physician.

Medical records are a combination of previous medical reports, self-reported patient information, as well as a physician's notes on diagnoses, care, and treatments. These histories also involve a variety of information about health, lifestyle and personal habits. A medical history interview helps your doctor understand not only yours but your family's medical history. We get most amused at the number of phone calls a patient makes to his/her spouse, parent or caregiver, as they realise they do not have adequate information about their medical history! So bring your spouse or a reliable relative for your doctor's appointment to report the medical history. There are questions that they might know best. For example, you may think you don't snore, or be less realistic about reporting details of your lifestyle choices.

Ensure that you have compiled the following:

- Records pertaining to significant illnesses and current or past medical conditions
- A list of current medications- and ensure your emergency contact is aware of this list
- Documentation on diagnostic laboratory test findings, diagnoses, and treatment plans
- Complete review of systems as a first-level check to determine baseline health, allergies, current medications, and any adverse reactions
- Records of preventive therapies such as immunisations and screenings
- Prescriptions and paperwork pertaining to services performed by medical professionals
- Discharge notes from previous hospitalisations, including details like dates, times, attending medical personnel's, prescriptions, and any other diagnostic data or lab reports

Furthermore, having blind faith that your primary care physician or family doctor knows it all and can provide information when needed, can prove to be dangerous. One of our members, Mr Jaggi Malhotra was visiting his son in New York, where he met with a severe car accident. A cab car driver supposedly had a seizure and lost control and his vehicle came right onto Mrs and Mr Malhotra at full speed. They survived this horrific accident and were lying on the floor, right outside the Apple store on Fifth Avenue, facing Central Park. Luckily, Mr Malhotra's son knew that he has a concierge physician who knew about all the medication his parents were taking, so he called us.

Not only did the TMC team know their medications, but the team alerted the emergency doctors about Mrs Malhotra's allergy to common prophylaxis and Sulphur, which is the first line of treatment for any accidents. We gave patient portal access to the son and to the emergency doctors on duty since we keep digitised medical records of all our clients. If this information was not shared with the doctors at the right time, the case could have gotten worse.

So it's important to keep up to date records of all previous scans, films and data. Further, a complete record includes information from three generations of relatives, including children, brothers and sisters, parents, aunts and uncles, nieces and nephews, grandparents, and cousins.

There are a number of conditions or diseases which are genetic or hereditary. If the family medical history is in place, the current symptoms can be linked to the conditions of your family members and any latent disease can be analysed and healed before it gets too late.

If you want to know how medical history can be helpful, refer to the last chapter of the book.

Rule # 4 – If technology has advanced, there is no reason for you to remain medieval

Are you using technology to your advantage? Where and how do you keep this critical data? Do you keep your financial records in one place? Does someone maintain them for you? A chartered accountant or a wealth manager? Who manages all your medical data? Do you even see the value in having medical data?

Until recently, all of this medical data was paper-driven. This format made the medical records vulnerable to various errors, loss and omission. Globally, there is a trend to keep it in an electronic form and they are now being digitised, which keeps them safe and also let you access them whenever and wherever you want. The human error quotient has been now minimised with instantaneous access to the information.

Keep your records accessible on the cloud in an electronic form. This will help you in the following ways:

- Providing a more organised approach towards healthcare
- Allowing the caregiver to grip the medical condition better and form a strong base for further investigation and treatment
- Facilitating a clear and smoother communication with other team members
- Meeting Legal and ethical obligations. The electronic records act as clear and legit records for hospitals, medical regulatory authorities (colleges) and legislative institutions
- Acting as a solid evidence: In case of conflict, it clearly reflects the events as they happened

"[1]In a recent review article by the Journal of the American Medical Informatics Association on patient access to medical records, it was found that 75 percent to 95 percent of patients were interested in enrolling in a patient-accessible medical record system. However, only 0.4 per cent of patients were found to submit spontaneous requests for their medical records under the current systems.

Low requests for medical records by patients are attributed to the onerous and often confusing process to obtain medical records through government pathways."

It is hence evident that improper medical records is a global issue and needs to be tackled with advanced technology that is available. Technology has advanced due to research and the United States is the Holy Grail for cutting-edge research. The world is far smaller than it used to be, thanks to technology.

In 2015, my mother in-law was detected with uterine cancer during a routine preventive test. In her case, the endometrial cancer cells had only invaded the muscle of the uterus and not the surrounding organs or lymph nodes, which indicates that the cancer had been caught at an early stage. However, the treatment and management plan provided to her in Delhi was a "radical total hysterectomy with lymph node dissection". This is an open surgery, meaning the abdominal surgical incision is 5-6 inches long, so that the uterus and lymph nodes can be removed through this incision. The Indian hospital told us that she would stay in hospital for 8 days have at least 3 different tubes sticking out of her body and oh yes, a ton of antibiotics would be administered to keep the hospital bugs at bay. Also the surgeon performing the surgery is a general surgeon who removes tumors from every part of the body – whether it be in the brain or in your toe.

Horrified by this, we then decided to consult a gynaecologist from St Lukes BCM at Texas Medical Center and we were given the option of consulting a gynaecologic oncology surgeon. After reviewing the case and the biopsy sample which was taken from India, she suggested a third option of using the Da Vinci Robot for the Hysterectomy. With the Da Vinci robotic instruments, you have a full view of the surgical field that allows for greater precision. This trumps the laparoscopic approach of limited visualisation and the open surgery approach of lesser precision. Along with these advantages, they also allow for:

1. Lesser bleeding and complications
2. Decreased infections
3. Reduced hospital stay
4. Lesser incisions
5. Better outcomes and healing

The world is more globalised, so taking advantage of medical advancements is a lot easier than it was back in the day.

Rule # 5 – Do understand your condition and treatment and act accordingly and do follow as prescribed

It has been further found out that,

"[2]Four out of five Americans who visit the doctor leave with a prescription. In 2007, more than 3.5 billion prescriptions were written, and that number is expected to grow to more than four billion by 2010."

But what is happening with these prescriptions? Are they being followed? It has been reported that three out of four Americans are not taking their medical prescriptions as per the directions provided. It is reported that:

- They tend to forget to take their medicines
- They don't fill the prescription
- They discontinue the course before it is finished
- Intake dosage which is less than what has been recommended so that the side effects can be avoided or the cost can be reduced

Many patients fail to understand their condition completely and are not sure about the treatment they are going to get for the same. Result – they are not able to work as a team with the doctor. If your doctor doesn't seem to understand what you are trying to say, repeat your symptoms using your own terms. This will help make sure your doctor gets the right diagnosis and develops the proper treatment.

To get the highest quality care, you must have your patient profile ready, which would include complete information about your condition, previous hospitalisations or any kind of surgeries that you had in past, and medications that you had been subjected to or any kind of allergies to medicine or food items. A detailed patient profile will help the doctor know your entire medical history, while none of the critical information is missed. A sample profile that we give all our members at TMC is appended in the last chapter for your reference.

Half of all American adults – 90 million people – have difficulty understanding and acting on health information. For India, the situation would be worse. But it's one thing that you are not capable of understanding. However, a number of people don't want to probe. They are in denial, have an emotional blockage or have God complex that no disease is powerful enough to have an impact on them. One of my staff members had diabetes, hypertension and obesity, but he was not ready to quit smoking. Working in a healthcare company and witnessing a number of cases on daily basis, he was still not able to get over his denial.

Who is a bad patient? A bad patient is someone who might not be following all the rules we are discussing here. A bad patient is someone:

- Who only talks about starting dieting because the physician suggested and doesn't take it seriously
- Who lies about his drinking, smoking and eating habits
- Whose is not having any preventive strategy
- Who is not taking his prescriptions and medications seriously
- Who thinks he/she should see a doctor only when he/ she is ill
- Who is not taking proper appointments
- Takes doctors for granted
- Anyone else who a doctor would like to fire

Rule # 6 – Don't take non-credible second opinions

According to a survey,

- 70 percent people take second opinion for home improvement
- 55 percent people take second opinion for car repair
- But only 23 percent people take second opinion for teeth straightening

Well, if you are like most of the Google geeks, you probably land up at a physician's office after diagnosing yourself. But halt for a minute to think about how you go about that Google search or that second medical opinion. Who suggested the second doctor? A friend, a relative, or a family doctor? What network, knowledge or experience does this person have? Is he/she someone who has studied all the medical history and found you the best specialist for that set of problems? How do you know that this specialist saw each and every piece of information that was needed? Is he/she the one who is able to join the dots?

- 35% of Americans have gone online to figure out a health problem
- Of those, 36% discovered they needed the help of a professional, while
- 38% found that they could take care of the problem themselves
- The numbers of those with chronic conditions who search for their problems online are even higher and approach 60%

Remember the case of breast cancer we discussed in the chapter – Medical Deity? A non-credible second opinion doesn't just mean that you are taking an opinion from another family member, relative, friend or colleague. An opinion becomes credible only when it comes from a professional who has proper understanding of your case and history. Otherwise, it's nothing more than a random shot in the dark which might very well come back and hit you; like it did to the patient in the case of breast cancer we discussed.

Every day in our practice, we come across people with a scatter gun approach to doctor shopping. Moreover, people are freely recommending doctors on Facebook, WhatsApp groups, blogs without even understanding the condition.

"Does anyone know a good oncologist?"

Come on! Is the general public a credible source for deciphering if you need a medical oncologist or an Onco surgeon? Today, oncology is such a diverse field that the specialists are limiting themselves to certain diseases and types of cancers only. How does your uncle, aunt or friend know this? Furthermore, unfortunately in India, we have an issue where more often than not you get a full course of treatment from the first doctor you go to.

Finding a good doctor is no more a challenge. In fact, every major city in the world now has good doctors who have shining degrees and badges. It is crucial to find the right good doctor who can be different for each patient.

Rule # 7 – Don't self-medicate because of ignorance, overconfidence or "Googleance"

According to a survey,

"[3]Eight out of ten adults self-medicate using over-the-counter (OTC) medicines for various health conditions in the past year, most often for colds, coughs and seasonal allergies. In a recent survey, many consumers say they turn to OTCs because of convenience and a desire to save time, money and a trip to the doctor."

It has been further found that one in five adults who self-medicate admit they have not used OTC medicines as directed, either by taking more than the recommended dose or by taking these medicines more frequently than indicated! Forget about getting healed, such immature attitude can push you further down the line.

Numerous prescriptions result in an amplified error. According to a study, more than 1.5 million Americans are victims of preventable medical errors per year. The complications are a result of:

- Intake of multiple medicines (also known as polypharmacy)
- Drug interactions
- Human error (unclear instructions, giving wrong dose or forgetfulness)
- Poor medical management (incorrect medication, lack of communication)

Patients take decisions in the absence of medical intelligence all the time. And I would like to pose the same question. Whom do you trust with your finances? A professional or anyone random who has no knowledge of finance? It is sad to see people who fail to realise that their health is the real wealth. They entrust individuals with their health, who might not have any medical intelligence.

Mrs Malhotra is the best living example of a self-medicating deity. She has got treatment for every minute or severe disease one might encounter in life. In fact she does not hesitate in prescribing medications to doctors. Once Mr. Malhotra was having problems with his sleep occasionally and she medicated him with a pill from her magic box of medicine. The process was repeated and eventually Mr. Malhotra realized his dependence on the pill to sleep. His body had developed an addiction to it!

Rule # 8 – Don't be a dinosaur

1. Communicate symptoms accurately

"Doctor sahib, he doesn't like my cooking anymore; does not like my family members. He eats only milk and cereal in the morning and he is not hungry from within and does not like to walk." That was my aunt – Mrs Bhatia, telling the medical condition of her husband to the doctor. So, she was emotional and shared what was disturbing her emotionally. In a Punjabi house, if you are eating – it means all is well. Everything revolves around food! But a doctor wants to hear something else when we use the term *medical condition*, something more specific perhaps. They want to know the exact symptoms and how the patient is feeling. The symptoms would help the doctor understand the case and prescribe accordingly. If you think you are not ready, you can prepare in advance before communicating. All you need to do is to be organised and figure out answers for the following questions:

- Why are you visiting the doctor?
- Any new symptoms since last week?
- Have things improved?
- Any other questions?

Keep your list short and focussed. If your list is too long, it might not highlight what is significant and must be communicated. There are many patients who don't mention a number of symptoms because they feel that it is a part of their personality. But every minute detail is important and can influence the interpretation of results that doctors would come up with.

2. Don't pretend to be clueless or exaggerate symptoms

Place facts accurately and don't act like a Zombie – clueless of everything happening to you. Also, don't exaggerate your symptoms. Doctor's sympathy is not going to heal you. It is the understanding of your precise medical condition that would help you get healed. Moreover, be serious when you visit your doctor.

> *"[4]If you're happily texting and laughing with your friends until the second you spot me walking into your room, I'm not going to believe that your pain is a ten out of ten."*

3. Don't display these annoying behaviours to doctors

While you visit your doctor, you have to make sure that your appointment is productive and efficient. Try not to annoy the doctor by doing the following[5]:

- Stinking feet or breath – bad hygiene
- Complaining about other doctors – bitching never helps
- Bombarding with questions outside clinic e.g. meeting at a grocery store or mall
- Asking too many question. The enthusiasm is well-appreciated but there is a limit

- Insulting or showing superiority to a staff member or a nurse – patient Superhero complex
- Providing self-diagnosis. Provide symptoms not the diagnosis. That is the doctor's job, he /she spent a decade studying medicine.
- Wandering while blabbing on your phone
- Overreacting

Rule # 9 – Understand your defense mechanisms

Analyse your behaviours and reactions to either doctors or to yourself. Psychologists talk about "defense mechanisms," or manners in which we behave or think in certain ways to better protect or "defend" ourselves.

As summarised by Dr Grehol, a defense mechanism is a way to look how individuals are moving far from a state of complete awareness of probable unpleasant thoughts, behaviours and their own fears. Everyone has a different way to handle difficulties and pain. And these different ways are the defense mechanisms which can be either healthy or unhealthy – depending upon how they are being used!

The categorisation of these defense mechanism is done by analysing how primitive the mechanisms are. The more primitive it is, the less effect it will have on the individual on a long-term basis; most of the primitive defense mechanism are short term and are found mostly in children. As far as adults are concerned, their primitive defense mechanisms are a result of stress or traumatic events.

Most of these psychological defense mechanisms are unconscious and individuals are not really aware that a defense mechanism is being used. Sometimes the use of these coping strategies makes people dysfunctional or ends up harming them. There are psychotherapy sessions which can make individuals aware of when they are using these behaviours. Almost all us deploy these coping mechanisms. Eventually, you can control these and learn to use less of the primitive ones, and rather, use more effective ones to your own advantage.

Name of Defense Mechanism	Description	Example
Repression	Suppressing a thought or desire in oneself so that it remains unconscious. It can also act as a ground for other defense mechanisms to grow upon	A man has a phobia of heights but cannot remember the first time he felt this fear
Denial	Not accepting reality because either it is too painful or you are not ready for it	You are diagnosed with diabetes but you refuse to accept it by saying it's borderline
Regression	Leading to the temporary or long-term reversion of the ego to an earlier stage of development, rather than handling unacceptable impulses in a more matured way	Each time someone mentions your obesity, you stomp off into another room and pout.

Projection	It is also known as blame shifting. When you deny some attributes in you and blame them to be present in the others	You get inherently angry at your doctor but subconsciously such anger is unacceptable, so you compensate by saying that the doctor is angry with you and is not offering the right treatment Note: "It's not me, it's you who feel that way towards me."
Displacement	Displacing the feeling from the original source and translating it into action through something else	When you get mad at your diagnosis, but you break your dinner plate by throwing them against the wall saying the food was horrible.
Reaction Formation	Adopting beliefs, attitudes, and feelings contrary to what you really believe	You say you are a homophobe while being homosexual yourself.
Rationalization	By giving fabricated justifications for irrational actions or feelings	"It was the patient's fault. If he wasn't so (obese, sick etc), this error wouldn't have caused so much harm."

Altruism	Handling your own pain by helping others	After your diagnosis you exhaust and drown yourself in volunteer work at your church.
Humor	Focussing on funny aspects of a painful situation	A person's treatment for cancer makes him lose his hair so he makes jokes about being bald or bald people.

Rule # 10 – Know yourself

Stop seeing yourselves merely as a body of flesh, blood and bones. You are more than that and you know it well. You are an amazing creation. Establish and realise a connection between your mind, body and soul. There is so much more to what we see and perceive by our limited senses. It's important to take responsibility and understand that the secret of health doesn't exist outside but inside you.

EIGHT

Superconscious Medicine

"Digital health is already here and in widespread use. But, stealing a famous line from novelist William Gibson, 'The future is already here – it's just not very evenly distributed.' The same holds true for digital health. It's already empowering us in a multitude of ways to manage and optimize our own health, and it's transforming and disrupting our healthcare systems and the manner in which we receive healthcare."

– Paul Sonnier-Founder, Digital Health Living.

The technological revolution has made consumerisation of health a reality. Patients are now empowered consumers who can demand answers and have complete rights to seek quality service. With smartphones, apps and the Internet, everything is just a click away. Everything can be managed in an efficient way, way beyond what we could have imagined a decade ago.

It is the era of Health 3.0, which will let individual access information that is tailored for him/her or derived from their electronic health records and other social network resources. This will ensure sorted out information which is exclusively modified for the individual. While most of the communication and exchange of information traditionally was verbal, through Ehealth, we can use Internet and electronic resources to enhance the communication and exchange information faster and effectively. Ehealth further has segmented to Mhealth which involves the use of mobile devices to collect and share the medical data and information even more conveniently.

Two unprecedented revolutions are underway, according to Gregory Stock:

The first is the silicon revolution involving all the telecommunications, computers and related technology that are reshaping our lives. We are taking silicon – the inert sand at our feet – and breathing into it a level of complexity that is beginning to rival life itself. We are animating the inanimate, and our world will never be the same. The second – a child of the first – is the revolution in genomics, and more broadly, molecular biology. We are unraveling the workings of life and beginning to shape our own evolutionary future.

While we have super-specialised doctors, it is time now that we must also have superconscious patients who are exposed to the concept of superconscious medicine. Take advantage of concierge medicine, which is the medicine of this digital era.

A superconscious patient is a proactive individual who experiences him/herself as a whole and is aware of all the aspects associated with his/ her holistic health, while using technology and every other viable resource available to him/her. A superconscious patient is the centre of the superconscious star.

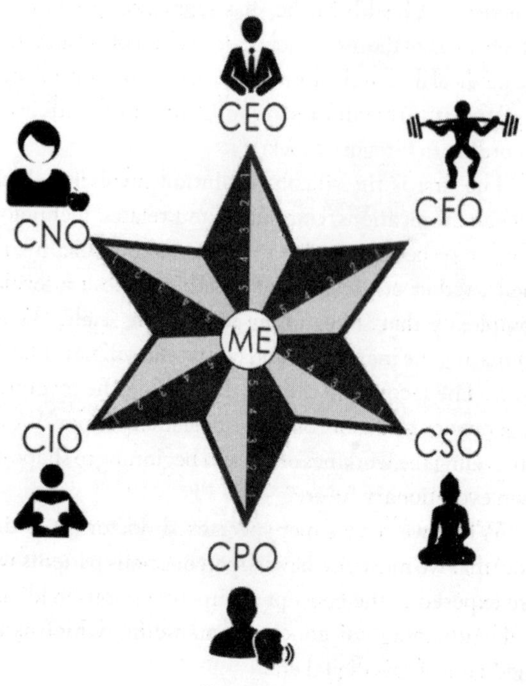

Illustration 3

The star is your lense for taking stock of your healthcare choices and awareness level. Take a moment to think what your star looks like. At each edge of the star, name the person that you have entrusted with a particular aspect of your health.

Who constitutes your healthcare team; not doctors who will take care of your sickness? When we fall sick, we have little control over the decisions we take, as often others have the final word.

CEO – Chief Executive Officer – Family doctor, concierge physician, spouse, parent

CSO – Chief Spiritual Officer – Guru, mentor, philosopher

CFO – Chief Fitness Officer – Physical trainer, yoga teacher, fitness partner

CNO – Chief Nutrition Officer – Nutritionist, health coach, chef, spouse

CPO – Chief Psychological Officer – Therapist, agony aunt, spouse, friend

CIO – Chief Intellectual Officer – Mentor, teacher, boss, role model

To get an analytical result of the status of your level of superconsciousness, follow the steps below:

1. Analyse the star. You can notice a series of numbers (1 to 5).
2. Further, assess yourself on the **F-SPINE Awareness** check. Rate yourself on how you are constantly growing in each aspect of the Superconscious

Star (fitness, spirituality, psychological well-being, intellectual growth, nutrition). The officer in-charge is the person who you have appointed to manage that aspect. The score will indicate the efficiency of your level of conscious choice.

Elements of F-SPINE	Officer In-charge	Score (1 to 5)
Fitness		
Spiritual Growth		
Psychological Well being		
Intellectual Growth		
Nutrition		
Executive empowered to take all medical decisions for you		

3. Plot these scores and connect the dots on the Superconscious Star.
4. Observe the figure.
5. Closer you are to the centre, the more aware and in control you are holistically. The rounder the figure is and the closer it is to the nucleus, the more conscious and centred you are.

Reflect on the choices you have made and think about your relationship with yourself. Evaluate why you have designated these roles to the people you have. You may not have actually thought of certain aspects and would've wanted to score a zero. But don't be so harsh on yourself;

no one deserves a zero as there is at least a little awareness somewhere.

Some Superconscious questions for Superconscious stars:

1. Which are the areas of the Superconscious Star that I need to work on?
2. Am I super organised with my medical data?
3. Do I have my SMART goals for health defined?
4. Do I have a preventive plan documented ?
5. Do I completely understand my existing medical conditions and their treatment, including side effects of medication?
6. Do I have a well defined healthcare support system and team?

To begin with, evaluate the role of your healthcare team:

CEO – Chief Executive Officer – Family Doctor, Concierge Physician, Spouse, Parent

- Develop a relationship with the client-build confidence and trust.
- Technology assisted medical data awareness.
- Coordination between various branches of healing.

CSO – Chief Spiritual Officer – Guru, Mentor, Philosopher

- Assists with finding solutions and answers based on a spiritual philosophy.

- Connects beliefs to health.
- Helps gain a deeper meaning of life and its challenges.

CFO – Chief Fitness Officer – Physical Trainer, Yoga teacher, Fitness partner

- Prevention and treatment – for injuries or physical conditions.
- Physical conditioning, strength training, exercise techniques.
- Mobility support and performance enhancement.

CNO – Chief Nutrition Officer – Nutritionist, Health Coach, Chef, Spouse

- Building body's immune response, metabolism rate, detox.
- Assessing food requirements and diet habits by lifestyle/personality type.
- Balance of nutrition during adverse condition – extreme stress like chemotherapy, burns, anxiety etc

CPO – Chief Psychological Officer – Therapist, Agony Aunt, Spouse, Friend

- Balance between mental and physical health
- Identifying somatic manifestations of psychological conditions
- Dealing with emotions associated with illness, support, and management of chronic illness.

CIO – Chief intellectual Officer – Mentor, Teacher, Boss, Role Model

- Helps with intellectual growth and balance by guidance and assistance with decision making, risks versus benefits etc.
- Outlines intellectual goals that help enhance your potential and wellbeing.
- Helps avoid taking on intellectual endeavors not suitable for you based on an in-depth understanding of individual potential and personality type.

It's important to reflect on a situation from different lenses so that you make an informed choice – the human body is very complex and we may think we have understood ourselves and have all the answers, but with technological advancement and evolution, I urge you to remain a seeker. Try and understand the spiritual significance of the situation you are in. Take it as a blessing or a learning experience.

Acceptance with a sense of objectivity is step one to raising your level of awareness. Try talking to yourself in second person to analyse a situation if you find it hard being objective.

Here is an example of how we do it at our medical concierge practice:

I follow the TMC nine-step approach that either helps me understand the cause or consider different treatments before acting.

At TMC, we follow the integrated medicine approach where experts from each field collaborate with each other and approach towards the holistic well-being of the patient. Our integrated medicine wheel is comprised of the elements shown below:

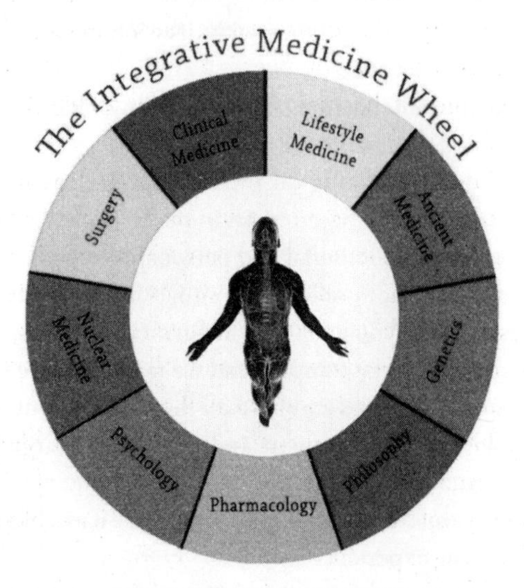

Illustration 4

Medical Condition: *Aanchal, you have chronic untreated Asthma which has led to bronchiectasis. Now you have a few options to reverse the condition or let it progress into a bigger disease.*

a. Clinical medicine – A pulmonologist and an asthma allergy specialist, both will help manage my conditions.
b. Pharmacology – my options are that I get on medication for the next four months.

c. Nuclear medicine – I need a CT scan, X ray, etc. to help me monitor further progression.
d. Genetics – There is a strong genetic cause for my asthma but no genetic cure.
e. Surgery – If I don't take care, there will be invasive bronchoscopies or other interventions that may be required if the disease progresses eventually, leading to a lung transplant.
f. Ancient medicine – Yoga, Ayurveda and naturopathy can help me make some lifestyle changes and surely help with prevention or further relapse, so I need to find a way to get my Ayurveda and clinical medicine treatment to align.
g. Lifestyle medicine – Naturopathy, diet, meditation and stress management will help me heal from within, find my inner balance and help identify triggers.
h. Psychology – Thoughts, behaviour and feeling. What is the secondary gain of having this disease? What emotional need is this sickness fulfilling?
i. Philosophy – I will look at spiritual answers to explain my present condition. So I believe that I am suffering from a lung condition so that I can make an impact through my not-for-profit, Breathe Easy India. I am meant to suffer so that I can heal.

I know this is very hard to do on your own. I am fortunate to have a team of specialists at TMC who actually help me. This is not just an Indian problem; the most popular example that I can think of is that of Steve Jobs who regretted not having a patient advocate or a designated health CEO. He faced problems that he could never imagine facing while running Apple Inc., which is the world's most valuable brand with a valuation of close to US$119 billion. His entire case is solid testimony to why you must appoint the CEO of your health. Sickness was a long journey for Jobs which lasted 11 years. Here is an excerpt from his biography which shows that there is a huge void that exists in the world of healthcare[1].

"The following Saturday afternoon (after bowing down to the inevitable that he may not ever go back to work, he announced to the Apple Board that he needed another medical leave and that Tim Cook should take charge of day-to-day operations), Jobs allowed his wife to convene a meeting of his doctors. He realised that he was facing the type of problem that he never permitted at Apple. His treatment was fragmented rather than integrated. Each of his myriad maladies was being treated by different specialists – oncologists, pain specialists, nutritionists, hepatologists, and hematologists – but they were not being co-ordinated in a cohesive approach, the way James Eason had done in Memphis. 'One of the big issues in the healthcare industry is the lack of caseworkers or advocates that are the quarterback of each team', Laurene Powell Jobs said. This was particularly true at Stanford, where nobody seemed in charge of figuring out how nutrition was related to pain care and to oncology."

Below is a chronology of events that he had to face because of not having a systematic and superconscious approach to his health, because he lacked that quarterback that focussed on integrating all systems for care and health.

Early 1990 – CT scan done to examine his kidneys and ureter, as he had developed recurrent kidney stones. The diagnosis of his cancer was actually serendipitous.

October 2003 – CT scan of his urinary system was repeated in five years where they found a suspicious lesion on his pancreas.

Pancreatic scan – He was referred for a pancreatic scan for detailed diagnosis. Suspicion made was of standard pancreatic adenocarcinoma, the deadly kind that few survive.

Transduodenal biopsy – The procedure confirmed the diagnosis of neuro endocrine tumour. He started searching naturopathic treatment and started a strict vegan diet with lots of juices, especially carrot and orange juices.

Aug 2004 – Jobs finally has his pancreatic tumour removed by surgery. It has been delayed by nine months.

2008 – Jobs lost 40lbs of weight due to higher levels of Glucagon as a result of his liver metastasis. He flew to Basel, Switzerland to try experimental hormone therapy. He also underwent experimental treatment developed in Rotterdam, known as peptide receptor radionuclide therapy.

Apr 2009 – Jobs receives a liver transplant at the Methodist University Hospital in Memphis, Tennessee.

November 2010 – Jobs' condition deteriorated; he was in pain, stopped eating, and had to be fed intravenously by a nurse.

Early 2011 – Doctors detected the recurrence that was causing these symptoms. Ultimately, he developed liver, bone, and other metastases and was in a lot of pain.

He starts to find targeted therapy for his cancer but ultimately resistance occurs and cancer prevails over the therapy.

October 2011 – Steve Jobs dies

While Steve Jobs was a revolution in the world of technology, the next revolution to have an equal impact on mankind according to Gregory Stock will be the merging of humans and machines in a global superorganism with the help of modern technology.

His intellectual breakthrough provides a powerful new way of looking at macro-evolution and interpreting the relationship between technology and biology, and of incorporating the modern hi-tech world into a biological framework.

Science and spirituality are aligning and if Professor Stock's philosophy holds true, then we are superorganisms which transcend humanity. Humans are special. We are unique. We need to awaken to some realities that exist at realms that seem disconnected on the face of it, but with a deeper look it's all interconnected and interrelated.

"[2]The next frontier is not space, but our own selves, and it is going to be quite a journey. He believes that

no consensus will emerge about the many possibilities being ushered in by today's revolution in genomics, proteomics, molecular biology and regenerative medicine. The developments speak too forcefully about who we are and what we will become. Our reactions to them depend too much on politics, religion, philosophy, history and values."

The time is right for us to start asking ourselves some fundamental questions which may seem radical today but will help us ride the change. The time is right for us to face ourselves and accept responsibility and take control of this beautiful gift of life.

NINE

Tips Tools and Rules

Functions of Family Doctor or Primary Care Physician:

1. Obtain your complete health history and perform physical examinations.
2. Maintain electronic health records.
3. Diagnose and direct counseling on a plan for treatment.
4. Prescribe medication for conditions in line with his/her expertise.
5. Perform minor surgical procedures.
6. Arrange referral for patients after thorough research and examination.
7. Make clinical summaries.
8. Review incoming reports (e.g. lab, x-ray, EKG) sign, date and follow-up in a timely manner.
9. Participate in peer review, quality assurance, provider meetings, and other clinical meetings.

10. Assist in updating protocols and principles of practice as requested.
11. Assist in outside medical public relations functions.
12. Supervise mid-level practitioners (physician assistants and nurse practitioners).
13. Impart medical advice upon consultation with International doctors and Houston Office Team
14. Manage the client scheduling with national/international doctors, service providers.

SAMPLE MEDICAL SUMMARY

MRN: 1000001083 Date: 15-Dec-2015

Dear Sir,

Greetings from Texas Medical Concierge!

Thank you for giving our medical concierge the opportunity to provide our advisory and consultancy services.

This is an Integrated Health Consultancy Report drafted by our medical team after reviewing your Medical Reports and Medical History.

This report:

1. Summarizes your medical conditions
2. Outlines your health goals
3. Highlights your risk factors
4. Recommends specialists for conditions that need to be monitored and evaluated.

OUR HEALTH MODULE

"Health is a state of complete physical, mental and social well-being and not merely the absence of disease or infirmity" (WHO).

We at Texas Medical Concierge believe that to achieve near perfect health it has to be through the integration of mind body and soul. We help you with setting your physical health goals and providing you all your modern medicine options through our cutting edge Tele-medicine technologies and collaborations with Global Centers of Excellence.

Further, we also guide you to align other aspects of Holistic Healing.

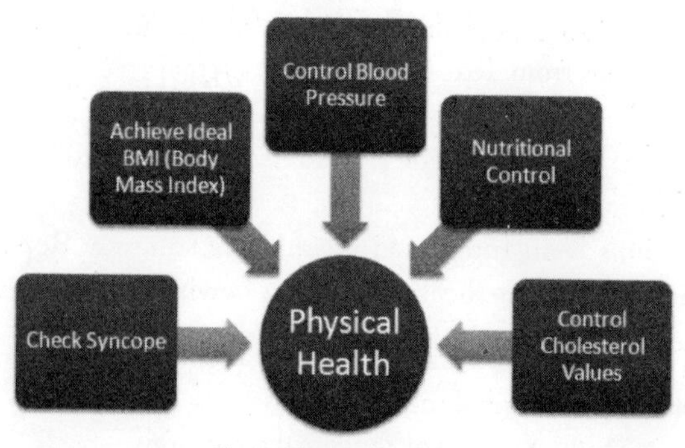

Physical Health Goals

EXISTING MEDICAL CONDITIONS

- Syncope
- Dyslipidemia
- Hypertension

PAST MEDICAL HISTORY

- Hernia repair Surgery (45 years back)
- Anal Fistula Repair Surgery (2013)
- B/L Cataract surgery (2013)
- Jaundice (2000)

The health conditions mentioned above are on the basis of signs, symptoms and investigation results which you have provided. If you would like to receive a medical second opinion for confirmation of diagnosis, we would be able to provide that to you from global experts.

CURRENT MEDICATIONS

1. Tab. Amtas (Amlodipine 5mg) – Once a Day

Amlodipine is in a group of drugs called calcium channel blockers. Amlodipine relaxes (widens) blood vessels and improves blood flow.

Uses:

Hypertension, Angina (chest pain) and it may even used to avoid myocardial infarction.

Side Effects:

Swelling in your hands, ankles, or feet, pounding heartbeats or fluttering in your chest, chest pain or heavy feeling, nausea, sweating, constipation and general ill feeling

2. Tab. Losartan 50 mg BD

Losartan is in group of angiotensin receptor blocker (ARBs). It works by relaxing blood vessels.

Uses:

Hypertension, prevent strokes and heart attacks.

Side Effects:

Dizziness or lightheadedness, cough, abdominal pain

3. Tab. Arvast (Rosuvastatin 5mg) OD

Rosuvastatin is a member of the drug class of statins, used to treat high cholesterol and related conditions, and to prevent cardiovascular disease.

Uses:

Decrease Cholesterol levels, prevent strokes and heart attacks.

Side Effects:

Headache, dizziness, constipation, nausea, vomiting, abdominal pain, myalgia, chest pain, peripheral edema, depression, insomnia, rash

4. Tab. Aspirin 75 mg OD

Aspirin has an anti-platelet effect by inhibiting the production of thromboxane, which under normal circumstances binds platelet molecules together to repair damaged blood vessels.

Uses:

Prevent heart attacks, strokes, and blood clot formation in people at high risk for developing blood clots.

Side Effects:

GI disturbances; prolonged bleeding time, rhinitis, urticaria and epigastric discomfort; tinnitus, bronchospasm

5. Tab. Neurocare (Vitamin B complex) OD

It is a Vitamin B complex supplement

Uses:

Diabetic, Alcoholic or Toxic neuropathies, Neuritis, Neuralgia, Cervical Syndrome, Shoulder-arm syndrome, Lumbago, Sciatica

Side Effects:

Allergic hypersensitivity reactions

6. Vitamin B 12 injection once a week

It is a Vitamin B supplement

Uses:

Diabetic, Alcoholic or Toxic neuropathies, Neuritis, Neuralgia, Cervical Syndrome, Shoulder-arm syndrome, Lumbago, Sciatica

Side Effects:

Allergic hypersensitivity reactions

7. Cap DV 60 k (Calcium Supplement) – OD

Uses:

Calcium supports the growth of strong bones and teeth. Calcium is the most plentiful mineral in the body and is essential in processes such as nerve transmission, intracellular signaling, hormonal secretion, and vascular and muscle function. It may reduce the risk of rickets and osteoporosis. Rich sources of calcium include dairy products, such as cheese, milk, and yogurt.

Side Effects:

Dietary calcium is generally safe, if the calcium in your diet and from supplements exceeds the tolerable upper limit, you could increase your risk of health problems, such as: Kidney stones, Constipation, Calcium buildup in your blood vessels, impaired absorption of iron and zinc.

BMI:

The body mass index (BMI), or Quetelet index, is a measure of relative size based on the mass and height of an individual. Your BMI is **27.97 kg/m²**.

Category	BMI range – kg/m2	BMI Prime
Very severely underweight	less than 15	less than 0.60
Severely underweight	from 15.0 to 16.0	from 0.60 to 0.64
Underweight	from 16.0.to 18.5	from 0.64 to 0.74
Normal (healthy weight)	from 18.5 to 25	from 0.74 to 1.0
Overweight	from 25 to 30	from 1.0 to 1.2
Obese Class I (Moderately obese)	from 30 to 35	from 1.2 to 1.4
Obese Class II (Severely obese)	from 35 to 40	from 1.4 to 1.6
Obese Class III (Very severely obese)	over 40	over 1.6

The first step to living well with the above mentioned problems is to understand them

SYNCOPE

Syncope, also known as fainting, passing out and swooning, is defined as a short loss of consciousness and muscle strength, characterized by a fast onset, short duration, and spontaneous recovery.

Sign & Symptoms

- Light headedness
- Tunnel vision – your field of vision is constricted so that you see only what's in front of you
- Nausea
- A cold, clammy sweat
- Blurred vision

Management

- **Specialist**: Neurologist, Cardiologist/Internal Medicine.
- **Medication**: None
- **Surgery**: Pacemaker can help if cardio aspect is ascertained.
- **Diagnostic Tests**: EEG, ECG, MRI/CT head, Stress Test, Head Up tilt test
- **Lifestyle & Rehabilitation**: Self-monitoring of weight, Consumption of a low-fat diet, Daily physical activity (Aerobic isotonic exercise) of approximately 60 minutes or an average of 300 minutes per week.

HYPERTENSION

Hypertension (HTN) or high blood pressure is a chronic medical condition in which the blood pressure in the arteries is elevated. Hypertension is diagnosed on the basis of a persistent high blood pressure.

Classification of Hypertension (JNC7)

Category	Systolic pressure	Diastolic pressure
Unit	mmHg	mmHg
Normal	90–119	60–79
High normal or Pre-hypertension	120–139	80–89
Stage 1 hypertension	140–159	90–99
Stage 2 hypertension	160-179	100-109
Stage 3 hypertension (Hypertensive emergency)	≥180	≥110
Isolated systolic hypertension	≥140	<90

Signs & Symptoms

Hypertension is rarely accompanied by any symptoms, and its identification is usually through screening. A proportion of people with high blood pressure complaints of Headache, Vertigo, Tinnitus, Altered vision or Fainting episodes.

Management

- **Specialist**: Endocrinologist, Internal Medicine, Nutritionist

- **Medication**: Thiazide diuretics, Beta blockers, Angiotensin-converting enzyme (ACE) inhibitors, Angiotensin II receptor blockers (ARBs), Calcium channel blockers, Renin inhibitors, Vasodilators, Aldosterone antagonists.
- **Surgery**: NA
- **Diagnostic Tests**: Blood pressure monitoring, fasting lipid panel, Liver function studies, thyroid function tests.
- **Lifestyle & Rehabilitation**: Eat healthy foods, decrease the salt in your diet, maintain a healthy weight, increase physical activity, limit alcohol, manage stress, monitor your blood pressure at home and practice relaxation or slow, deep breathing.
- **Preventive**: Healthy diet, regular exercise.

DYSLIPIDEMIA

Dyslipidemia is elevation of plasma cholesterol, triglycerides (TGs), or both, or a low high-density lipoprotein level in the blood that contributes to the development of atherosclerosis.

Signs & Symptoms

Dyslipidemia is usually asymptomatic until cholesterol levels are greater than 200mg/dL. Patients may report pain, which is commonly mid epigastric but may occur in other regions, including the chest or back.

Management

- **Specialist**: Internist/ Cardiologist/ Endocrinologist
- **Medication**: Statins (Niacin/ fibrates combination), Bile-acid-binding resins, Cholesterol absorption inhibitors, Omega Acids
- **Surgery**: LDL apheresis, Ileal bypass, Liver transplantation, Portocaval
- **Diagnostic tests**: Lipid Analysis, Apoprotein B
- **Lifestyle & Rehabilitation**: Program of progressive aerobic and toning exercise, weight loss, and dietary management can significantly lower triglyceride levels and, in some cases, normalize them
- **Preventive**: Quit Smoking, Restrain alcohol drinks to not more than one per day (for male), Eat a low-fat, low-salt diet that includes many fruits, vegetables and whole grains

HIGH RISK CONDITIONS

The values below signify the number of positive risk factors you have.

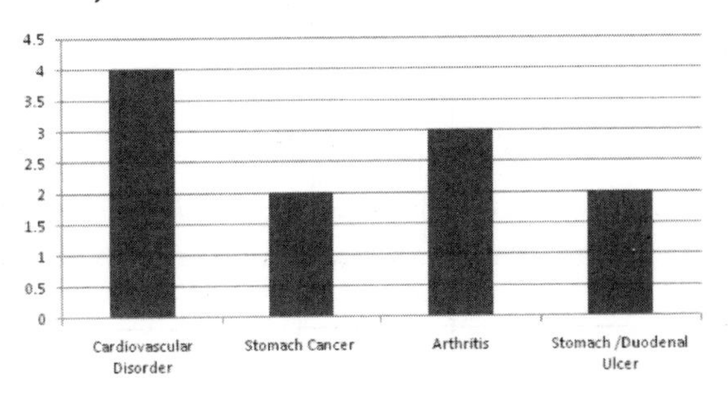

OUR RECOMMENDATIONS TO HELP YOU MEET YOUR HEALTH GOALS

1. Getting preventive care is one of the most important steps you can take to manage your health. When a condition is diagnosed early, it is usually easier to treat, thus regular checkups can help identify lifestyle changes you can make to avoid progress of disease.

General Screening	Investigations	Frequency
Bone and Joint Study	Serum. Vitamin D3 Bone Mineral Density	Every Six Months After 12 Months
Hematology Study	– Haemoglobin – White Blood Cell Count – Differential Count – Red Blood Cell Count – Haematocrit – Red Cell Indices (MCV, MCH, MCHC) – Red Cell Distribution Width – Platelet Count – Peripheral Blood Film – Erythrocyte Sedimentation Rate (ESR)	Annually

Kidney Study	– Sodium – Potassium – Chloride – Bicarbonate – Urea – Phosphorous – Calcium – Creatinine – eGFR -BUN – Uric Acid	Annually
Liver Study	Total Bilirubin – Direct & Indirect Bilirubin – Total Protein – Albumin – Globulin – SGOT/SGPT – Alkaline Phosphatase – GGT	Annually
Lipid Profile	– Total Cholesterol – HDL Cholesterol – LDL Cholesterol – Triglycerides – Cholesterol/HDL Ratio – Apo lipoprotein B	Annually
Urine Analysis	– Urine Routine/ Microscopic Examination	Annually

Stool Analysis	– Stool Routine/ Occult Blood	
Diabetes Study	HbA1c Fasting Glucose Glucose tolerance test	Annually Once

RADIOLOGY INVESTIGATIONS

Cardiac Study	TMT with Echo, 24-Hrs Holter Monitoring Head up-Tilt Test	Once
Abdomen & Pelvis	Esophageal Manometry, Endoscopy Colonoscopy	Once
Neurology	MRI Head and Spine Screening	Once

Vitals	Blood Pressure Weight	Daily Monthly

2. A consultation with a Dr. XYZ or Dr ABC for current stage risk assessment, preventive steps and also use of medical therapy for management of conditions above.
3. Further please keep your medical history handy or contact your concierge physician who is fully aware of your medical history.

How complete Medical History can help:

- It helps to be fully aware of the medications the patient has, makes self administration more effective.
- It helps to identify and document allergies a particular substance and is valuable information in emergency situations. It helps to determine the proper first aid for a person depending on his/her medical conditions and medications he/she is taking. Different people might need different treatments for the same cause due to variance in medical history.For instance, if a person allergic to bee is stung by a bee, you will have to give him/her a treatment different from the normal one.
- It helps to respond to emergencies the right way, as quickly as possible. By keeping an easily accessible medical history sheet for a particular person, you will be able to share it with emergency personnel without wasting valuable time – time which may determine life or death.
- It helps to properly respond to newly developed symptoms. Depending on a person's medical history, you will be able to determine whether these symptoms are a result of an illness that has already been diagnosed or if they are a part of a new condition. For example, if a person is known to have frequent bouts of migraine, you can administer medications accordingly. But if a person who has never been diagnosed of migraine complains about recurrent severe headaches, you may have to get a set of diagnostic tests done or see certain specialists.

Metaphysical significance of Body Parts

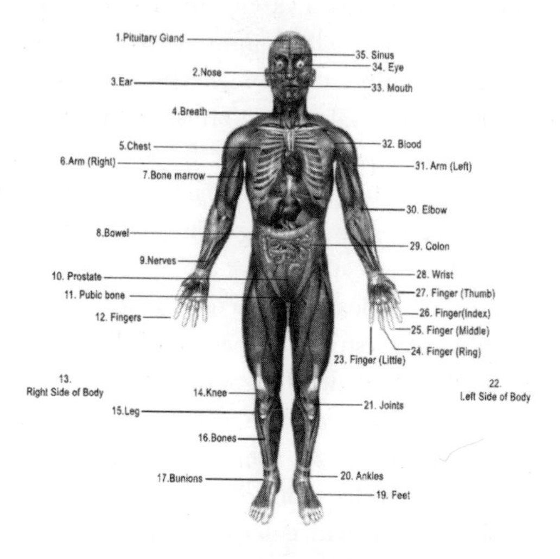

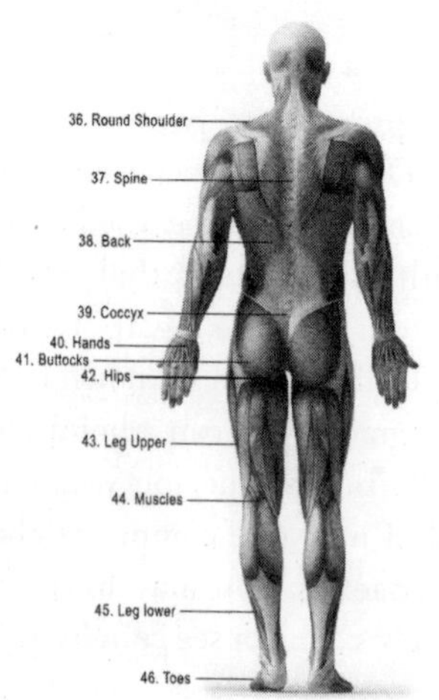

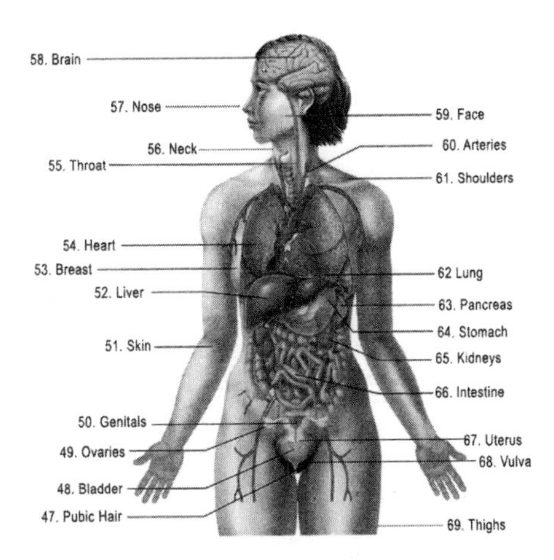

1. *Pituitary Gland* – Represents the control center. Feeling out of control, or not in control of your own destiny.
2. *Nose* – Represents self-recognition.
3. *Ear* – Indicates how you interact with your environment and your ability to listen.
4. *Breath* – Represents the ability to take in life.
5. *Chest* – A lack of compassion. Not feeling that your emotions are valid or considered.
6. *Arm (Right)* – Signifies Giving.
7. *Bone marrow* – Represents deepest beliefs about the self. How you support and care for yourself.
8. *Bowel* – Represent the release of waste.
9. *Nerves* – Represent communication and sensitivity towards a situation not acknowledged in conscious mind.
10. *Prostate* – Represents the masculine principle.
11. *Pubic bone* – Represents protection.
12. *Fingers* – Represent the detail of life.
13. *Right Side of Body* – Masculine energies, giving, putting out, the "do side", or physical side. Men, or father.
14. *Knee* – Represents pride and ego.
15. *Leg* – Carry us forward in life.
16. *Bones* – Represents the structure of your life.
17. *Bunions* – Represents lack of Joy in meeting experiences in life.
18. Nails – Represent protection.
19. *Feet* – Represent our understanding – of ourselves, of life, of others.
20. *Ankles* – Represents our support system and flexibility.
21. *Joints* – Represent changes in direction in life and the ease of these movements.
22. *Left Side of Body* – Represents receptivity, taking in, feminine energy, women, the mother.
23. *Finger (Little)* – Represents the family and pretending. Ignoring your own creativity, or issues with linking to family.
24. *Finger (Ring)* – Represent the details of life.
25. *Finger (Middle)* – Represents anger and sexuality.
26. *Finger (Index)* – Represents ego and fear. Fear of authority, or egotistical; abusing your authority.

27. *Finger (Thumb)* – Represents intellect and worry. Worry, always thinking. Being under someone's thumb.
28. *Wrist* – Represents Stability movement, congruency, integrity and grace.
29. *Colon* – Fear of letting go. Holding on to the past.
30. *Elbow* – Represents changing directions and accepting new experiences.
31. *Arm (Left)* – Signifies Receiving.
32. *Blood* – Represents joy in the body, flowing freely. Circulation of ideas.
33. *Mouth* – Represents taking in of new ideas and nourishment. Set opinions. Closed mind. Incapacity to take in new ideas.
34. *Eye* – Represents the capacity to see clearly past, present, future.
35. *Sinus* – Represents confusion.
36. *Round Shoulder* – Carrying the burden of life. Helpless and hopeless.
37. *Spine* – Flexible support of life.
38. *Back* – Represents Support.
39. *Coccyx* – Represents the fundamental needs
40. *Hands* – Represents the holding on or letting go.
41. *Buttocks* – Represents power. Loose Buttocks, loss of power.
42. *Hips* – Represents balance. Fear of going forward in major decisions. Nothing to move forward to.
43. *Leg Upper* – Holding on to old childhood traumas.
44. *Muscles* – Resistance to new experiences. Muscles represent our ability to move in life.
45. *Leg lower* – Represent moving forward, taking action getting started.
46. *Toes* – Represents the minor details of the future.
47. *Public Hair* – Represents both attraction and hiding. Neither children nor the elderly have pubic hair.
48. *Bladder* – Represents the emotional resistance to life.
49. *Ovaries* – Represent points of creation. Creativity. Inability to express or accept your own creativity.
50. *Genitals* – Represent the masculine and feminine principles. Worry about not being good enough.
51. *Skin* – Represents our Individuality. Represents how we present ourselves to the world, as a reflection of how we see ourselves.
52. *Liver* – Liver is the seat of anger, primitive emotions and rage.
53. *Breast* – Represents mothering and nurturing and nourishment.
54. *Heart* – Represents the center of love and security.
55. *Throat* – Avenue of expression. Channel of Creativity.
56. *Neck* – Represents inflexibility or stubbornness.
57. *Nose* – Represents self-recognition.
58. *Brain* – Represents the computer, the switchboard.
59. *Face* – Represents what we show the world.
60. *Arteries* – Carry the joy of life.
61. *Shoulders* – Represents our ability to carry our experiences.
62. *Lung* – The ability to take in life. Depression. Grief. Not feeling worthy of living life fully.
63. *Pancreas* – Represents the sweetness of life.
64. *Stomach* – Holds nourishment. Digests ideas.
65. *Kidneys* – Holding on to anger or resentments.
66. *Intestine* – Assimilation. Absorption, elimination with ease.
67. *Uterus* – Represents the home of creativity.
68. *Vulva* – Represents Vulnerability.
69. *Thighs* – Our ideals, confidence and power. It also represents new beginnings and forward movements.

Ailments and their Metaphysical causes

**The research on this list is still ongoing and the list is evolving to be more accurate. To find the updated list, visit www.aanchalbhatia.com

Name of Ailment	*Metaphysical Reason*	*Also see*
Abdominal Cramps	Fear. Stopping the process. Refusal to flow with experiences.	Pain
Abscess and revenge.	Fermenting thoughts over hurts, slights Boils	Infections,
Accidents	Inability to speak up for the self. Rebellion against authority. Belief in violence. Anger.	trauma, injuries
Aches	Longing for love. Longing to be held.	pain
Acne	Not accepting oneself. Dislike of self	Skin, Pimples
Addictions	Running from the self. Inability to face fear. Not knowing how to love oneself, self-rejection	Alcoholism

Addison's disease	Severe emotional malnutrition. Anger at the self	
Adenoids	Family friction arguments. Child feeling unwelcome or in the way.	Tonsillitis
Adrenal Problems	Defeatism. No longer caring for the self. Anxiety.	
Ageing Problems	Fear of being one's self. Rejection of social beliefs. Old thinking.	
AIDS	Feeling defenseless and hopeless. Nobody cares. A strong belief in not being good enough. Denial of the self. Sexual guilt.	Infection, Immuno-logic
Alcoholism	Feeling of futility, guilt, inadequacy. Self rejection. Running away from responsibilities.	Addictions
Amnesia	Running from life. Inability to stand up for the self.	
Anemia	Lack of joy. Fear of life. Not feeling good enough	Blood
Ankle Problems	Represents mobility and direction, acknowledgement of the emotions associated with this change of lifestyle. Inflexibility and guilt associated with adapting to change.	Arthritis
Anorexia	denying the self & life. Extreme fear, self hatred and rejection.	Loss of Appetite
Anorectal bleeding (Hemato-chezia)	Anger and frustration, irritability, stress, resentment, depression,	Anemia, Anus

Anus (Hemorr-hoids)	Issues with dumping and releasing, extreme excitation of emotions	anorectal bleeding, pain
Anus (Abscess)	Anger in relation to what you don't want to release.	abscess, Infections, pain
Anus Fistula	Incomplete releasing of trash. Holding on to garbage of the past.	abscess, Infections, pain, Fistula
Anus Itching (Pruritus Ani)	Guilt over the past. Remorse. Blocking the flow of good.	fissure and hemorr-hoids
Anus Pain	Guilt. Desire for punishment. Not feeling good enough	Pain
Anxiety/ Nervous-ness	Distrust, Not trusting the natural flow of life.	
Apathy	Resistance to feeling. Deadening of the self.	
Appetite (excessive)	Needing protection. Judging your own emotions	Obesity
Appetite (Loss of)	Protecting the self. Not trusting life.	
Arterios-clerosis	Resistance, Tension. Hardened narrow-mindedness. Refusing to see good.	Heart
Arthritic Fingers	A desire to punish. Blame. Feeling victimized.	Hand, Joints
Arthritis	Feeling unloved. Criticism, Strong resentments.	Joints.

Asphyxiating Attacks	Breathing problems, Hyperventilation. Fear. Not trusting the process of life. Getting stuck in childhood.	Respiratory, Obstructive
Asthma	Unresolved guilt. Smother love. Inabilty to breath for one's self. Feeling stifled. Suppressed crying.	Respiratory ailments, Lungs, Allergies, Chronic Disease
Asthma (Babies & Children)	Fear of life. Not wanting to be here.	Respiratory ailments, Lungs, Allergies
Allergies	Sustained feelings of being out of control, Irritation with life. Chronic need to please others	
Alzheimer's Disease	Refusal to deal with the world as it is. A desire to leave the planet.	Amnesia
Athlete's Foot	Frustration at not being accepted. Inability to move forward with ease	Bones
Back Issues	Lack of emotinal support or feeling unloved	Pain, Spine, Bone Problems
Back Problems: – Rounded shoulders	Carrying the burdens of life. Helpless and hopeless, holding on to dissapointment	Spine, Arthritis, Pain
Back Pain (Upper)	Lack of emotional support. Feeling unloved. Holding back love.	Spine, Arthritis, Pain, Back issues

Back Pain (Mid)	Guilt. Stuck in all that stuff back there. Wanting to get the pressure off or someone to back off	Spine, Arthritis, Pain, Back issues
Back Pain (Lower)	Financial woes and concerns. Fear of money. Lack of financial support.	Spine, Arthritis, Pain, Back issues
Bad Breath	Anger and revengeful thoughts. Experiences backing up.	Mouth Problems
Balance Issues (loss of)	Scattered thinking. Not centred.	
Baldness	Fear. Tension. Trying to control everything and not trusting in the process of life.	
Bedwetting	Fear of parent, usually the father.	
Bites	Fear. Open to every slight.	
Bite (Animal)	Anger turned inward. A need for punishment.	Rabies
Bug Bite	Guilt over small things.	
Blackheads	Small outbursts of anger. Feeling Dirty and Unloved	Comedones
Birth defects	Karmic. You selected to come out that way to learn or teach lessons. We choose our parents. Dealing with unfinished business.	
Belching	Gulping life too quickly, absorbing other peoples energy	
Bell's Palsy	Extreme control over anger. Unwillingness to express feelings	

Bladder Problems	Anxiety. Holding on to old ideas. Fear of letting go. Being "pissed off"	Prostate
Bleeding Gums	Lack of joy in the decision made in life.	Teeth, Gum Problems
Bleeding	Joy running out. Anger	Blood
Blisters	Resistance. Lack of emotional protection	Skin, Infections
Blood Pressure: – High	Longstanding emotional problem not solved.	Heart, Chronic Disease
Blood Pressure – Low	Lack of love, and defeatism. A helpless attitude in life	Heart, Chronic Disease
Bone Problems	Mental pressures and tightness. The structures of life/universe.	
Break/ Fractures	Rebelling against authority	
Bone Deformity	Mental pressure and tightness. Muscles can't stretch. Loss of mental mobility.	
Bowel Problems	Not letting go of the old feeling no longer needed.	
Bright's Disease	Feeling like a kid who can't do it right and is not good enough. Sense of failure. Loss.	
Brain Tumor	Incorrect computerized beliefs. Stubborn. Refusing to change old patterns.	
Breast Problems (Left)	Feeling unloved, refusal to nourish oneself. Putting everyone else first.	

Breast Problems (Right)	Over protection, over bearing, difficulty in giving love.	
Breast Lumps	A refusal to nourish the self. Putting everyone else first. Over mothering. Overprotection. Overbearing attitudes	
Breathing Problems	Not trusting the process of life. Getting stuck in childhood. Fear of taking in life fully. Fear or refusal to take in life fully. Not feeling the right to take up space or even exist.	Respiratory ailments, Asthma, Lungs
Bronchitis	Inflamed family environment. Arguments and yelling. Sometimes silent family discord.	Respiratory ailments, Asthma, Lungs
Bruises	The little bumps in life. Self-punishment.	
Blood Problems	Lack of joy. Lack of circulation of ideas.	
Blood Clotting	Closing down the flow of joy.	
Boils	Anger. Boiled over. Seething. Rebellion	Pimples, Abseces
Bulimia	Hopeless terror. A frantic stuffing and purging of self-hatred	
Burns	Anger. Burning up. Incensed	
Bunions	Lack of joy in meeting the experiences of life.	Bones
Bursitis	Repressed anger. Wanting to hit someone	Joints

Bruxism	frustration regarding your self-expression result of holding back what you want to express and achieve in your life.	Jaw Problems
Calluses	Hardened concepts and ideas. Fear solidified	Corns, Foot Problems
Cancer	Deep hurt. Longstanding resentment. Something is eating you up within, Deep secret or grief eating away at the self. Carrying hatred.Strong feelings of abandonment, betrayal and fear of being alone.	Chronic disease
Candida	Feeling very scattered. Lots of frustration and anger. Demanding and untrusting in relationships. Overactive and unsatisfied mind	Fungus, Infection
Canker Sores	Festering words held back by the lips. Blame, scarred within	Infections, Abscess
Car Sickness	Bondage. Feeling of being trapped. Anxiety, grief, or other emotions can also cause motion sickness.	Motion Sickness
Carbuncle	Poisonous anger about personal injustices.	Boils, Absceses
Carpal Tunnel Syndrome	Anger and frustration at life's seeming injustices and stresses	Nerve, Neurology
Cataracts	Inability to see ahead with joy. Dark future	Eyes
Cellulite	Stored anger and self-punishment	Hormonal, Metabolic
Cerebral Palsy	A need to unite the family in an action of love	Mental Health

Chills	Mental contraction, pulling away inwards and desire to retreat	Fever, Cold
Cholesterol	Clogging the channels of joy. Fear of accepting joy	Endocrine, Liver, Metabollic, Obesity, Cardio-vascular
Chronic Disease	A refusal to change. Fear of the future. Not feeling safe.	
Circulation	Represents the ability to feel and express the emotions in positive ways	Blood
Cold Sores (Fever Blisters)	Festering angry words and fear of expressing them.	Burns
Colds (Upper Respiratory illness)	Too much going on at once. Mental confusion, disorder. Small hurts	Respiratory
Colic	Mental irritation, impatience, annoyance in the surroundings	Behaviour
Colitis	Insecurity. Represents the ease of letting go of that which is over. Over-exacting parents. Feeling of oppression & defeat. Great need for affection.	
Coma	Fear. Trying to escape from something or someone.	
Comedones	Small outbursts of anger.	Blackheads
Conjunc-tivitis	Anger and frustration at what you are looking at in life	Eyes

Consti-pation	Incomplete releasing. Holding on to garbage of the past. Guilt over the past. Sometimes stinginess. Refusing to release old ideas. Stuck in the past	
Corns	Hardened areas of thought – stubborn holding on to the pain of the past.	Calluses, Foot Problems
Coronary Thrombosis	Feeling alone & Scared. Not good enough. Don't do enough. Will never make it.	
Cushing's Disease	Mental imbalance. Overproduction of crushing ideas. A feeling of being overpowered.	
Coughs	A desire to bark at the world. "Listen to me!"	
Cramps	Tension. Fear. Gripping, holding on	
Crohn's Disease	Fear. Worry. Not feeling good enough	
Cuts	Punishment for not following your own rules.	
Cysts	Running the old painful movie. Nursing hurts. A false growth.	
Cystic Fibrosis	A thick belief that life won't work for you. "Poor me."	
Cavities	When you do not make a plan to achieve what you want in life, your mind recycles the same information without any output. Therefore, you continosly mull over the same thoughts in your mind and they start to 'eat away' at you. You need to put your ideas into action in order to keep progressing.	Teeth

Deafness	Rejection, stubbornness, isolation. What don't you want to hear? "Don't bother me."	Ear
Dementia	A refusal to deal with the world as it is. Hopelessness and anger	Alzheimer's Disease
Depression	Anger you feel you do not have a right to have. Hopelessness.	
Diabetes	Longing for what might have been. A great need to control. Deep sorrow. No sweetness left. Burdended with the struggles of life	Chronic Disease
Diarrhea	Fear and rejecting. Running off or away from something/someone.	
Dizziness	Flighty, scattered thinking. A refusal to look your fears or anxiety.	Vertigo
Dry eyes	Angry eyes. Refusing to see with love. Would rather die than forgive. Being spiteful.	Eyes
Dysentery	Fear and intense anger.	
Dysentery Amoebic	Believing they are out to get you.	
Dysentery Bacillary	Oppression and hopelessness	
Dysmeno-rrhea	Anger at the self. Hatred of the body or of the woman.	Menstrual Problems
Ear Problems	Not wanting to hear. Anger or too much turmoil and household arguments	
Eczema	Breath-taking antagonism. Mental eruptions.	Skin
Edema	Holding on and not letting go. What or who won't you let go of?	

Elbow Problems	Not being flexible, not able to change directions or accept new experiences.	Elbow
Emphysema	Fear of taking in life. Not worthy of living.	Lungs, Breathing and Respiratory Ailments
Endometriosis	Insecurity, disappointment and frustration. Replacing self-love with sugar. Blaming.	Uterus
Epilepsy	Sense of persecution. Rejection of life. A feeling of great struggle. Self-violence.	Seizures
Epstein-Barr Virus	Pushing beyond one's limits. Fear of not being good enough. Draining all inner support. Stress.	Viral, Mononucleosis
Eye (Astigmatism)	"I" trouble. Fear of really seeing the self.	
Eye (Hyperopia)	Fear of the present	
Eye (Myopia)	Fear of the future.	
Eye (Crossed)	Not wanting to see what's out there. Crossed purposes.	
Eyed Wall	Fear of looking at the present, right here	
Eye Problems (Children)	Not wanting to see what is going on in the family.	
Fainting	Fear. Can't cope. Blacking out what's really going on.	
Fatigue	Resistance, boredom. Lack of love for what one does.	Weakness

Flu (Influenza)	Responding to mass negativity. Putting too much faith in statistics.	Viral Infections
Fat or Weight issues	Oversensitivity. Often represents fear and shows a need for protection. Fear may be a cover for hidden anger and a resistance to forgive. Running away from feelings. Insecurity, self-rejection and seeking fulfillment.	Appetite (excess), obesity
Fat Belly	Anger at being denied nourishment	
Fat Hips	Lumps of stubborn anger at the parents.	
Fat Thighs	Packed childhood anger. Often rage at the father.	
Foot Problems	Fear of the future and of not stepping forward in life.	Corns, Callus
Fever	Anger. Burning up.	
Fibroid Tumors & Cysts	Nursing a hurt from a partner. A blow to the feminine ego.	Cancer
Food Poisoning	Allowing others to take control. Feeling defenseless.	Diarrhoea, Vomiting
Frigidity	Fear. Denial of pleasure. A belief that sex is bad. Insensitive partners. Fear of father.	
Fungus	Stagnating beliefs. Refusing to release the past. Letting the past rule today.	
Gallstones	Bitterness. Hard thoughts. Condemning. Pride.	
Gangrene	Mental morbidity. Drowning of joy with poisonous thoughts.	

Gas Problems	Gripping. Fear. Undigested ideas or concerns.	Abdominal cramps, Pain, Indigestion
Gastritis	Prolonged uncertainty. A feeling of doom.	Inflamm-ation
Gland Problems	Represent holding stations. Holding yourself back.	
Gout	The need to dominate. Impatience, anger.	Joints, Arthritis
Glaucoma	Stony unforgiveness. Pressure from longstanding hurts. Overwhelmed by it all.	Eye
Gray Hair	Stress. A belief in pressure and strain.	
Growths	Nursing those old hurts. Building resentments.	
Glandular Problems	Poor distribution of get up and go ideas. Holding yourself back.	
Goiter	Hatred for being inflicted upon. Victim. Feeling thwarted in life. Unfulfilled.	Hyper-thyroidism, Hypo-thyroidism
Gonorrhea	A need for punishment for being a bad person.	Venereal Disease
Gum Problems	Inability to back up decisions. Indecisive about life. Being wishy-washy about life.	Teeth
Halitosis	Rotten attitudes, vile gossip, foul thinking.	
Hand Problems	Grasping on to tight, not wanting to let go. Not 'handling' things well.	Hand

Hay Fever	Emotional congestion. Fear of the calendar. A belief in persecution or self denial. Guilt, Allergy to someone who denies you power	Allergy
Headaches	Invalidating the self. Self-criticism. Fear	Migraine Headaches
Heart Attack	Squeezing all the joy out of the heart in favor of money or position. Feeling alone and scared. "I'm not good enough. I don't do enough. I'll never make it."	Arterios-clerosis
Heart Problems	Longstanding emotional problems. Lack of joy, dealing with issues from anger, not love. Hardening of the heart. Belief in strain and stress.	Heart
Heartburn	Fear. Clutching onto fear. Not trusting in the process of life.	indigestion
Hepatitis	Resistance to change. Fear, anger, hatred.	Liver
Hernia	Ruptured relationships. Strain, burdens, incorrect creative expression.	
Herpes Genitalis	Mass belief in sexual guilt and the need for punishment. Public shame. Belief in a punishing God. Rejection of the genitals.	Viral Infections
Herpes Simplex	Bitter words left unspoken. Burning to bitch.	Viral Infections
Hip Problems	Fear of going forward in major decisions. Nothing to move forward to	Joints, Arthritis
Hirsutism	Anger that is covered over. The blanket used is usually fear. A desire to blame. There is often an unwillingness to nurture the self.	

Hives	Small, hidden fears. Mountains out of molehills.	Eczema, Urticaria
Hodgkin's Disease	Blame and a tremendous fear of not being good enough. A frantic race to prove one's self until the blood has no substance left to support itself. The joy of life is forgotten in the race of acceptance.	Cancer
Hunting-ton's Disease	Resentment at not being able to change others. Hopelessness.	
Hyper-thyroidism	Rage at being left out.	Gland Problems
Hypo-thyroidism	Giving up. Feeling hopelessly stifled.	Gland Problems
Hyper-activity	Fear. Feeling pressured and frantic.	
Hyper-ventilation	Resisting change. Not trusting the process. Resisting change. Not being able to take it all in.	
Hypo-glycemia	Overwhelmed by the burdens in life.	
Ileitis	Fear. Worry. Not being good enough.	Bowel Problems, Inflamation
Impotence	Sexual pressure, tension, guilt. Social beliefs. Spite against a previous mate. Fear of mother.	Frigidity
Inconti-nence	Emotional overflow. Years of controlling emotions.	Bladder Problems

Indigestion	Gut-level fear, dread, anxiety. Griping and grunting. Dread or anxiety about a recent or upcoming event	Heart Burn, Gas Problems
Infection	Irritation, anger, annoyance.	
Inflamm-ation	Seeing red. Inflamed thinking. Anger and frustration about conditions you are looking at in your life.	
Influenza	Response to mass negativity and beliefs. Fear. Belief in statistics.	Viral Infections
Ingrown Toenail	Worry and guilt about your right to move forward.	
Injuries	Anger at the self. Feeling guilty.	Accidents, Trauma
Insanity	Fleeing from the family. Escapism, withdrawal. Violent separation from life.	
Insomnia	Fear. Not trusting the process of life. Guilt.	
Itching – Pruritis	Un-satisfaction, having desires that go against the grain."Itching to get out."	Skin
Jaundice	Internal and external prejudice. Unbalanced reason.	Liver, Anemia
Jaw Problems	Anger. Resentment. Desire for revenge. Not letting go.	Teeth
Kidney Problems	Criticism, disappointment, failure. Shame. Reacting like a child. Feeling like you didn't do enough.	
Kidney Stones	Lumps of undissolved anger.	
keratitis	Extreme anger. A desire to hit those or what you see.	Eyes

Knee Problems	Stubborn ego and pride. Inability to bend. Fear. Inflexibility. Won't give in.	Joint, Arthritis
Laryngitis	So mad you can't speak. Fear of speaking up. Resentment of authority.	Sore Throat
Leprosy	Inability to handle life at all. A long held belief in not being good enough or clean enough.	Skin, Nerve
Liver Problem	Chronic complaining. Justifying fault-finding to deceive yourself. Feeling bad.	
Lockjaw	Anger. A desire to control. A refusal to express feelings.	Tetanus
Lump in the Throat	Fear. Not trusting the process of life.	Tumour Asthma, respiratory Ailments
Lung Problems	Depression, grief or fear of life. Not feeling worthy.	Asthma
Leucorrhea	A belief that women are powerless over the opposite sex anger at a mate.	Menstrual Problems
Leukemia	Brutally killing inspiration. What's the use?	Cancer
Lupus	A giving up. Better to die than stand up for one's self. Anger and punishment.	Skin, Joint
Lymph Problems	A warning that the mind needs to be recentered on the essentials of life. Love and joy.	
Malaria	Out of balance with nature and with life.	
Mastoiditis	Anger and frustration. A desire not to hear what is going on. Usually in children. Fear infecting the understanding	Ear, Pain, Deafness, Headache
Menopause Problems	Fear of no longer being wanted. Fear of aging. Self-rejection. Not feeling good enough.	

Menstrual Problems	Rejection of one's femininity. Guilt, fear. Belief that the genitals are sinful or dirty.	Dysmen-orrhea
Mental Problems & Senility	Returning to the "safety" of childhood. Demanding care and attention.	
Migraine Headaches	Sexual fears, or fear of being close, letting someone in too close. Feeling driven or pressured.	
Miscarriage	Fear of the future. Inappropriate timing.	
Mono-nucleosis	Anger at not receiving love and appre-ciation. No longer caring for the self.	Viral Infections
Motion Sickness	Fear. Bondage. Feeling of being trapped.	
Mouth Problems	Represents taking in of new ideas and nourishment. Set opinions. Closed mind. Incapacity to take in new idea	Pyorrhoea
Multiple Sclerosis	Mental hardness, hard-heartedness, iron will, inflexibility.	
Mucus Colon	Layered deposits of old confused thoughts clogging the channel of elimination. Wallowing in the gummed mire of the past	Crohn's Disease
Nail Biting	Frustration. Eating away at the self. Spite of a parent.	
Narcolepsy	Can't cope. Extreme fear. Wanting to get away from it all. Not wanting to be here.	
Nausea	Fear. Rejecting an idea or experience.	Food Poisoning

Neck Problems	Refusing to see other sides of a question.	Stubbornness, inflexibility. Unbending stubbornness.
Nephritis	Overreaction to disappointment and failure.	
Nervous Breakdown	Self-centeredness. Jamming the channels of communication.	
Nervousness	Fear, anxiety, struggle, rushing. Not trusting the process of life.	
Neuralgia	Punishment for guilt. Anguish over communication.	Pain
Nodules	Resentment and frustration and hurt ego over career.	Skin
Nose Bleeds	Crying out for love and recognition	
Nose (Runny)	Asking for help. Inner crying.	Allergy, Viral
Nose (Stuffy)	Not recognizing the self-worth.	
Numbness	Withholding love and consideration. Going dead mentally.	
Osteomyelitis	Anger and frustration at the very structure of life. Feeling unsupported.	Bone
Osteoporosis	Feeling there is no support left in life. Mental pressures and tightness. Muscles can't stretch. Loss of mental mobility.	Bone, Arthritis

Overweight	Fear, need for protection. Running away from feelings. Insecurity, self rejection. Seeking fulfillment.	Fat, Obesity
Pain	Guilt. Guilt always seeks punishment.	
Paralysis	Paralysing thoughts. Getting stuck. Terror leading to escape from a situation or person. Resistance.	Bell's Palsy, Stroke
Pancreas Problems	Not being able to enjoy the sweetness in life	
Pancreatitis	Rejection. Anger and frustration because life seems to have lost its sweetness.	Alcoholism
Parasites	Giving power to others, letting them take over and life off of you.	Malaria
Parkinson's Disease	Fear and an intense desire to control everything and everyone.	
Peptic Ulcer	Fear. A belief that you are not good enough. Anxious to please.	Gastritis
Phlebitis	Anger and frustration. Blaming others for the limitation and lack of joy in life. Emotional pain from past experiences that has not yet been released	
Pimples	Small outbursts of anger. See yourself as imperfect.	Skin, Acne
Pink Eye	Anger and frustration. Not wanting to see	Infection
Pneumonia	Desperate. Tired of life. Emotional wounds that are not allowed to heal.	Infection, Lung Problems
Poison Ivy	Allergy Feeling defenseless and open to attack.	Rash, Allergies

Polio	Paralysing jealousy. A desire to stop someone.	Viral
Post Nasal Drip	Inner crying. Childish tears. Victim.	
Premens-trual Syndrome	Allowing confusion to reign. Giving power to outside influences. Rejection of the feminine processes.	
Prostate Problems	Mental fears weaken the masculinity. Giving up. Sexual pressure and guilt. Belief in aging.	Urinary Infections
Psoriasis	Fear of being hurt. Deadening the senses of the self. Refusing to accept responsibility for our own feelings.	Skin
Pain	Pain represents emotional guilt, tension, and fear of moving forward.	
PMS (Pre-menstrual Syndrome)	It is a result of having conflicting emotions and resentment about being a female; unwilling to flow with nature. Allowing confusion to reign. Giving power to outside influences.	
Psoriasis	It represents excessive fear of being hurt due to damage to self-esteem in the past. Psoriasis is also associated with self-hatred and the belief that you are not worthy of being loved.	
Pubic Bone	Represents protection.	
Pyorrhoea	Anger at the inability to make decisions. Wishy-washy people.	Mouth Problems
Quinsy	A strong belief that you cannot speak up for yourself and ask for your needs	Tonsillitis

Quiver (Shake)	Feeling hopeless, can't regain control of one's life	
Rabies	Anger. A belief that violence is the answer.	Viral, Bite (Animal)
Respiratory Ailments	Fear of taking in life truly	Pneumonia
Rheuma-tism	Feeling victimized, lack of love or chronic bitterness.Resentment.	
Rheumatoid Arthritis	Deep criticism and authority. Feeling very put upon.	Arthritis, Joints
Rickets	Emotional malnutrition. Lack of love and security.	Arthritis
Root canal	Can't bite into anything anymore. Root belief being destroyed.	Teeth
Rash	Irritation over delays, attention seeking. Immature way to get attention.	Skin, Eczema
Ringworm	Allowing others to get under your skin. Not feeling good enough or clean enough.	Skin
Sagging lines	Sagging lines on the face come from sagging thoughts in the mind. Resent-ment of life.	Skin
Scabies	Infected thinking. Allowing others to get under your skin.	Skin, Rash
Sciatica	Being hypocritical. Fear of money and of the future	Spine Problem, Pain
Sclero-derma	Protecting the self from life. Not trusting yourself to be there and to take care of yourself	Skin

Scoliosis	Round shoulders, Spinal curvature.	Spine
Scratches	Feeling life tears at you, that life is a ripoff. That you are being ripped off	Skin
Sea sickness (motion Sickness)	Fear of death. Lack of control	
Seizures	Running away from the family, from the self or from life.	Epilepsy
Senility (Alzhei-mer's Disease)	Returning to the so called Safety of childhood. Demanding care and attention. A form of control of those around you. Escapism.	Dementia
Shin(s) Problems	Breaking down your ideals. Not living up to your own standards, or not being able to meet your standards. Setting your standards too high	
Shingles (varicella)	Waiting for the other shoe to drop. Fear and tension. Too sensitive	Viral Infection, Rash
Shoulders (joints rounds & shoulders)	Represent our ability to carry out experiences in life joyously. We make life a burden by our attitude.	
Shoulder Problems	Carrying the weight of the world on your shoulders. Feeling like life is a burden.	Arthritis
Sickle cell anemia	A belief that one is not good enough that destroys the very joy of life.	Blood
Sinus Problem (Sinusitis)	Irritation to one person, someone close. Chronic sinus infections represent the suppression of intuition	

Skin problems (Hives, psoriasis, rash)	Anxiety, fear. Old buried guck. I am being threatened.	Eczema
Slipped disc	Feeling totally unsupported by life	Back Pain, Spine Problem
Snoring	Stubborn refusal to let go of old patterns	Breathing Problems
Sore throat (Quinsy, Throat, Tonsillitis)	Holding in angry words. Feeling unable to express the self	Infection
Sores	Unexpressed anger that settles in	Ulcers
Spasms	Tightening our thoughts through fear. I release all restrictions, and I am free to be me.	Pain
Spastic Colitis (Colitis, Colon, intestines, mucus colon)	Fear of letting go. Insecurity	
Spinal Meningitis	Inflamed thinking and rage of life	
Spine Problem	Not feeling a flexible support of life	
Spleen	Obsessions. Being obsessed about things	

Sprains	Anger and resistance. Not wanting to move in a certain direction of life.	Pain
Sterility	Fear and resistance to the process of life, or not needing to go through the parenting experience	
Stiff Neck (neck problems)	Unbending Bull-headedness	Sprains, Pain
Stiffness	Rigid, stiff thinking	
Stomach Problems (Gastritis, heartburn, Peptic Ulcer, Ulcers)	Dread. Fear of the new. Inability to assimilate the new.	
Stroke (cerebro-vascular accident/ CVA)	Giving up. Resistance. ' rather die than change'. Rejection of life.Insecurity, lack of self-expression. Not being allowed to cry.	Paralysis
Stuttering	Insecurity. Lack of self expression. Not being allowed to cry.	
Sty (Eye problems)	Looking at life through angry eyes. Angry at someone.	Boils, Pain
Suicide	See life only in black and white. Refusal to see another way out.	
Swelling (Edema, Holdings fluids)	Being stuck in thinking. Clogged painful ideas.	

Tumors	Nursing old hurts and shocks. Building remorse.	Cancer
Tuber-culosis	Wasting away from selfishness. Possessive. Cruel thoughts. Revenge.	Infections, Lung Disorder
Teeth Problems	Being indecisive, not being able to break down ideas for analysis and decisions.	Cavities
Testticles Problems	Not accepting masculine principles, or the masculinity within.	
Thyroid Problems	Humiliation. Feeling repressed or put down. Feeling as if you never get to do what you want.Frustration around the inability to express oneself emotionally is a root cause of this illness. People who tend to be to nice.	Goitre, Hypothy-roidism, Hypert-hyroidism
Tonsillitis	Fear. Repressed emotions. Stifled Creativity.	
Thrush (Vaginal Infections)	Feeling sexually abused or exploited. Feelings of guilt, shame or repressed sexual feelings, or being intimate with the wrong person.	Mouth Problems
Throat Problems	The inability to speak up for oneself. Swallowed anger. Stifled creativity. Refusal to change.	Tonsillitis, Lump
Tapeworm	Strong belief in being a victim & unclean. Helpless to the seeming attitudes of others.	Infections
Tetanus	A need to release angry festering thoughts.	Lock Jaw, Spasm

Tinnitus	Refusal to listen. Not hearing the inner voice. Stubbornness. Tinnitus is an indication of intolerance to your environment which creates frustration.	Ear
Trauma	Stress, Extreme emotions	Accidents, injuries
Urethritis	Angry emotions. Being pissed off. Blame.	Pain
Ulcers (heartburn, Peptic ulcers, stomach problems)	Fear. A strong belief that you are not good enough.	
Urinary infections	Pissed off, usually at the opposite sex or a lover. Blaming others.	
Urticaria	energy of Discouragement in the emotional dimension.	Skin, Hives, Rash
Vaginitis	Anger at a mate. Sexual guilt. Punishing the self.	
Venereal Disease (AIDS, Gonorrhea, herpes, Syphilis)	Sexual guilt. Feeling a need for punishment. A belief that sexual intimacy is a sin or dirty.	
Varicose veins	Standing in the situation you hate. Discouragement. Feeling overworked and overburdened.	
Viral Infections	Lack of joy flowing through life. Living through bitterness.	

Varicose Veins	Standing in a situation you hate. Discouragement. Feeling over-worked and overburdened.negetive thinking, stress and numerological pressure or blockage	
Vertigo	Flighty, Scattered thinking. A refusal to look.	Dizziness
Vitiligo	Feeling completely outside of things. Not belonging. Not one of the group.	Skin
Vomiting	Violent rejection of ideas. Fear of the new.	Food Poisoning, Gastritis
Warts	Little expressions of hate. Feeling or believing you're ugly.	Viral, Skin
Warts (Plantar)	Anger at the very basis of your under-standing. Spreading frustration about the future.	
Whiteheads	Hiding ugliness	See comadones and blackheads
Weakness of body	A need for mental rest	Fatigue
Wounds	Anger and guilt at the self	Trauma, Injuries
Wisdom tooth impacted	Not giving yourself mental space to create a firm foundation.	Teeth
Wrist Problem	Not being flexible on an issue or situation. Not handling things with ease. Stubbornness.	Pain, Arthritis Wrist

Xenophobia	Fear of acceptance, feeling unworthy or fear of rejection,poor upbringing or alienation from people and cultures different than one's own.	
Yeast infections	Denying your own needs. Not suppor-ting yourself and busy taking care of others, unfinished buisiness, chronic psychological stress	Fungus
Zoophobia	Fear of accepting life's gifts and joys.	

References

CHAPTER 2

Source for Illustration 1: **http://www.bestmedicaldegrees.com/evolution/**

1. http://www.arunachala-ramana.org/forum/index.php?topic=6289.0

CHAPTER 3

1. http://www.ourcivilisation.com/medicine/usamed.htm
2. https://www.linkedin.com/in/idoweinberg
3. http://www.kevinmd.com/blog/2012/04/money-influences-decisions-doctors.html
4. http://www.ncbi.nlm.nih.gov/books/NBK61963/
5. http://www.simpletoremember.com/articles/a/einstein/

6. http://www.forbes.com/sites/matthewherper/2013/08/11/the-cost-of-inventing-a-new-drug-98-companies-ranked/
7. https://www.washingtonpost.com/news/wonk/wp/2015/02/11/big-pharmaceutical-companies-are-spending-far-more-on-marketing-than-research/
8. http://www.who.int/bulletin/volumes/88/4/10-010410/en/
9. https://www.kpmg.com/SG/en/IssuesAndInsights/ArticlesPublications/Documents/Advisory-Healthcare-3-Helping-organizations-unlock-the-value-of-big-data.pdf
10. http://www.nytimes.com/2006/02/22/business/22leonhardt.html?_r=0
11. http://www.indiaspend.com/sectors/rampant-corruption-just-one-challenge-in-indias-healthcare-struggle-53144
12. https://orfmumbai.wordpress.com/2014/10/17/corruption-in-indias-health-sector-begin-with-the-reform-of-medical-education/
13. http://www.nytimes.com/2006/02/22/business/22leonhardt.html?_r=0
14. http://www.ncpa.org/sub/dpd/index.php?Article_ID=23148
15. http://www.lifeextension.com/magazine/2004/3/awsi_death/page-04
16. http://www.webdc.com/pdfs/deathbymedicine.pdf
17. http://articles.mercola.com/sites/articles/archive/2000/07/30/doctors-death-part-one.aspx

CHAPTER 4

1. http://www.amazon.com/Youngest-Science-Medicine-Watcher-Alfred-Foundation/dp/0140243275/ref=pd_bbs_sr_4?ie=UTF8&s=books&qid=1224534386&sr=8-4
2. https://www.psychologytoday.com/experts/nassir-ghaemi-md-mph
3. https://www.psychologytoday.com/blog/mood-swings/200810/god-syndrome
4. http://www.halcyon.com/jmashmun/npd/dsm-iv.html
5. http://www.thecrimson.com/article/1973/4/27/professionalism-and-the-god-syndrome-pbobnly/
6. http://www.nytimes.com/2011/09/28/opinion/dowd-decoding-the-god-complex.html?_r=0
7. http://www.nytimes.com/2011/10/09/books/review/your-medical-mind-by-jerome-groopman-and-pamela-hartzband-book-review.html
8. http://medscape.typepad.com/thedifferential/2007/01/why_do_surgeons.html
9. http://forums.studentdoctor.net/threads/god-complex.436978/
10. http://medscape.typepad.com/thedifferential/2007/01/why_do_surgeons.html
11. http://www.imdb.com/title/tt0107497/quotes
12. http://www.nytimes.com/2007/04/01/books/review/Crichton.t.html
13. https://www.psychologytoday.com/blog/mood-swings/200810/god-syndrome

14. http://medscape.typepad.com/thedifferential/2007/01/why_do_surgeons.html
15. http://news.bbc.co.uk/2/hi/7654432.stm

CHAPTER 5

1. http://www.ipi.org.in/texts/others/pulkitsharma-sciencespirituality.php
2. Holocaust of attachment

CHAPTER 6

1. http://www.kevinmd.com/blog/2012/12/physicians-doctors-patients.html
2. http://www.drkevincampbellmd.com/
3. http://www.gmc-uk.org/doctorswhoarepatientsjanuary2010.pdf_62126868.pdf
4. http://www.healthcarebusinesstech.com/millennials-hospitals/
5. http://www.theguardian.com/society/2014/may/16/why-doctors-hide-their-own-illnesses
6. https://www.ache.org/policy/doctornursebehavior.pdf
7. https://www.medicalcouncil.ie/Information-for-Doctors/Good-Professional-Practice/
8. http://www.theguardian.com/society/2014/may/16/why-doctors-hide-their-own-illnesses
9. http://www.forbes.com/sites/robertpearl/2014/04/10/how-will-boomer-gen-x-millennial-doctors-respond-to-health-care-changes/

10. http://docplayer.net/9795504-Bad-blood-doctor-nurse-behavior-problems-impact-patient-care-by-carrie-johnson.html
11. https://www.medicalcouncil.ie/Information-for-Doctors/Good-Professional-Practice/
12. https://www.bostonglobe.com/magazine/2015/04/25/what-doctor-can-learn-from-being-patient/Sc3CDqv7yg1a2kvAFf2yeL/story.html
13. http://www.healthcarebusinesstech.com/millennials-hospitals/

CHAPTER 7

1. https://medchart.ca/Home/About
2. http://www.learnaboutrxsafety.org/healthy-dose.aspx
3. http://www.learnaboutrxsafety.org/healthy-dose.aspx
4. http://www.rd.com/health/conditions/50-secrets-your-nurse-wont-tell-you/
5. http://www.rd.com/health/conditions/annoying-patients/

CHAPTER 8

1. Steve Jobs by Walter Isaacson
2. http://www.gregorystock.net/philosophy.asp